Marion Frank

AIDS Education through Theatre

Case Studies from Uganda

Bayreuth African Studies 35

Dissertation der Fakultät Sprach- und Literaturwissenschaften
an der Universität Bayreuth

Die Deutsche Bibliothek - CIP-Einheitsaufnahme

Frank, Marion:
Aids education through theatre : case studies from Uganda /
Marion Frank. - Bayreuth : Bayreuth African Studies
Breitinger, 1995
(Bayreuth African studies series ; 35)
Zugl.: Bayreuth, Univ., Diss.
ISBN 3-927510-37-8
NE: GT

WG: 33;49 DBN 94.326532.0 95.01.12
7242 wi

D 703

Table of Contents

ACKNOWLEDGEMENTS

While working on this dissertation I received assistance, advice and support from a number of people and wish to acknowledge their contributions:

I would like to thank my *Doktorvater* Dr. habil. Eckhard Breitinger. My indebtedness to him will be evident throughout this work for developing the approach I have taken, and for patiently listening and discussing the draft with me at its various stages.

For advice, stimulating criticism and understanding I thank Professor Richard Taylor. His attitude encouraged and motivated me throughout my studies at Bayreuth University.

Special recognition goes to Claus Melchior whose friendship, advice, guidance, and encouragement was so important during the creation of this dissertation.

I am indebted to my friends whose friendship and counsel sustained me during the completion of this work: among those whom I would like to mention are Susanne Fendler, Michael Schön, Jürgen Jakobi, Gudrun Föttinger. I wish to thank Annette Urban for discussing parts of earlier drafts with me.

I cannot thank Ute Fendler and Jean-Claude Naba enough for their continuous friendship and assistance.

I am grateful to Lloyd B. Wilson for his assistance during my research in Uganda, and for tirelessly proof-reading the dissertation at its various stages. I also thank him for numerous stimulating and thought-provoking discussions and conversations.

A large part of the research for this dissertation was done in Uganda and Nigeria, and I want to thank all the people there who supported me and made me feel at home with their friendship and assistance:

I am particularly grateful to Professor Rose Mbowa from Makerere University in Kampala (Uganda) for her friendship, advice, as well as her numerous kindnesses and courtesies. I relied on her keen insight and interpretations of political and social events in Uganda to help understand the implications and challenges for the theatre.

I would like to mention Jessica Kaahwa, Vicky Owens, William Wagaba, Rainer and Alja Epp, Augustine Bazaale, Peter Lwanga, Axel T. Paul, Ron Kassimir in Uganda for their various contributions, as well as Jürgen Martini, Femi Osofisan, Olu Obafemi, Chris Dunton, Steve Oga Abah in Nigeria.

Friedrich-Naumann-Stiftung sponsored this dissertation for two and a half years - I would like to express my gratitude.

Last, but not least, I wish to thank my parents. Their support and encouragement have been without measure.

1. INTRODUCTION

1.1. Context of the Study

Towards the end of the 1970s, after three decades of development politics, the fact could no longer be ignored that many development-projects carried out during those 30 years had failed, and the need for new concepts became obvious. Inevitably, these projects were designed and implemented by Western planners who had arrived with preconceived notions of progress and how it was to be achieved while at the same time paying little attention to socio-cultural conditions in the target communities. Instead, economic growth was a fundamental consideration in all projects. By the late seventies, however, an awareness of the limits of purely economic approaches grew. In his address at the Third Committee of the United Nations General Assembly, Makaminian Makagiansar admitted that even though economic growth constitutes a basic factor of development, "the real yardstick of development is the extent to which it satisfies the socio-cultural needs and aspirations of individuals and communities."[1] This insight gave rise to new theoretical approaches and different paths of development which allowed the integration of a people's culture and history into the development process. Makagiansar stressed that cultural values determined the identity of a people, and they can become ideal tools "in a conscious effort to affect changes that societies wish to introduce in the interpretation of their past, in their organisational life and in their outlook on the future."[2]

One category of projects emanating from this line of thought included the use of theatre - which is the topic of this study. Government organisations (GOs), non-government organisations (NGOs) and international organisations (IOs) increasingly rely on theatre as an instrument for development. They seek to avoid the failures of the big and purely economically oriented development projects, by taking into account the socio-cultural background of target communities, thus acknowledging the existence of cultural diversity and plurality. Ideally, a play that is concerned with a certain problem and its solution, is created by members of

---

1 Makaminian Makagiansar, Assistant Director-General of UNESCO for Culture and Communication in 1978, in *Cultures*, Vol VI (Paris: The UNESCO Press and la Baconniere, 1979), pp. 11-15.

2 Makagiansar, p. 12.

the target group themselves. This, however, is only the case with purely project-oriented plays that are performed to implement a concrete improvement in the life of the community, as for example the building of a borehole. The plays which are the subject of this study do not belong to that category. Rather than dealing with concrete development aims, they are concerned with issues that call for a change of attitude within the target community, e.g. health education, environmental care et al. The solution to those problems requires expertise from outsiders, such as for instance medical doctors and nurses. Even though the factual information comes from outside, by using traditional theatre forms and having community members participate in the productions, the producers ensure the suggested solution is in accordance with the life and cultural values in the community. Among critics, theatre practitioners, and development workers, there exist various names for this kind of theatre: development theatre, theatre for development, popular theatre, community theatre, participatory theatre, theatre for the people, people's theatre.[3] While this form of theatre doubtlessly uses popular theatre traditions to convey messages, the terms popular theatre and theatre for the people still do not adequately describe the phenomenon. Similarly, community and participatory theatre are insufficient labels since they only refer to one aspect of this kind of theatre, i.e. its participatory character. In my opinion, Theatre for Development (TFD) is a more precise term, since it implies the notion that its primary concern is the promotion of development in a specific community - albeit through the use of popular theatre.[4] Another problem occurs when trying to determine the meaning of the term popular. One definition sees it in contrast with high or literary theatre. This distinction is based on linguistic and theatrical considerations. It follows Ngugi wa Thiongo's assumption that truly popular theatre is conducted in indigenous African languages whereas

---

3 Tar Ahura, "Popular and Participatory Theatre for Conscientization: the Question of Methodology," in *Practice of Community Theatre in Nigeria*, ed. Iyorwuese Harry Hagher (Jos: Society of Nigerian Theatre Artists (SONTA), 1990); Musa Dauda Enna, "Popular Theatre as a Tool for Socialist Emancipation," in *Practice of Community Theatre*, ed. I.H. Hagher; Chris Nwamuo, "Rural Development in Nigeria: The Community Theatre Paradigm," in *Practice of Community Theatre*, ed. I.H. Hagher; Ahmed Yerima, "Producing a Play for the Popular Theatre: a Study in Style and Technique in Samaru Projects," in *Practice of Community Theatre*, ed. I.H. Hagher; Iyorwuese Harry Hagher, "The Practice of Community Theatre for Development. Some Basic and non-Basic Contradictions," in *Practice of Community Theatre*, ed. Iyorwuese Harry Hagher.

4 I use the term TFD for both project-oriented plays and plays for consciousness raising.

theatre in foreign languages plays to an elite audience and is un-African.[5] Other critics define it according to aesthetic criteria such as literary form, or according to its mass appeal. Sandra Richardson, for example, calls Femi Osofisan a populist playwright and accordingly describes her notion of a populist theatre as one "which has a mass appeal, and so must necessarily build upon some of those aesthetic forms or structural patterns which a mass audience values."[6] As Desai and Cooper both remark, there is ambiguity in the notion of the term popular: is it defined by its choice of language, its mass appeal, or its relevance to the people? In "Popular Arts in Africa," Karin Barber refers to the usual definition that views popular art as opposed to traditional and elite art forms. Frederick Cooper draws attention to the fact that she equates the ambiguities inherent in the definition with those discovered by social scientists studying populism, and he concludes that "the difficulty with identifying the "populace," the "people," or the "masses" as a category is that it does not necessarily correspond to any particular relationship to the means of production, to any particular cultural characteristics, or to any set of aspirations, defintions of self, and set of relationships."[7] Other critical questions to pursue in this context are, as Cooper suggests, whether some art forms in Africa have specifically working class audiences; when did they develop and in relation to what social processes; and if the kind of social space created in African cities in the twentieth century has allowed for the development of boundary-crossing art forms in a particularly rich way. He points out that traditional art forms are varied and complex, and that the contradictions implicit in the modern notion of popular defining itself vis-à-vis elites may apply to an earlier, precolonial era. Those, as yet unanswered, questions point to some of the problems when trying to define the popular arts, since such a definition implies the need to discuss "the nature of the populace, and to stress the ambiguous definition of the producers and the audience of such artistic expression is to recognise the inchoate, uncertain, changeable nature

5 Gaurav Desai, "Theatre as Praxis: Discursive Strategies in African Popular Theatre," *African Studies Review*, Vol. 33, no. 1, April 1990, p. 66; Ngugi wa Thiong'o, *Decolonising the Mind: the Politics of Language in African Literature* (London: J. Currey, 1986).

6 Desai, "Theatre as Praxis," p. 66; Sandra Richards, "Toward a Populist Nigerian Theatre: The Plays of Femi Osofisan," *New Theatre Quarterly*, 3/11, 1987, pp. 280-88.

7 Frederick Cooper, "Who is the Populist?" *African Studies Review*, Vol. 30, no. 3, Sept. 1987; Karin Barber "Popular Arts in Africa," *African Studies Review*, Vol. 30, no. 3, September 1987.

of urban African society."[8] It seems that popular theatre cannot be defined in any one way. It is important to keep in mind, however, that it is in dialogue with other theatrical practices of a society, and that it arises from and constantly interacts with other modes of social discourse.[9] For the purpose of this study, which seeks to describe some popular theatre events in Africa and put them in relation to TFD in Uganda, Ross Kidd's definition seems to describe the phenomenon very aptly:

> As a means of expression which has traditionally been used to educate the young, unify the community, and articulate the commonly felt concerns and aspirations of the people... popular theatre builds on an educational approach and means of communication which is already familiar to and accepted by the community. It is their spontaneous means of education and grassroots communication.[10]

TFD projects try to go beyond the theatrical event. They want to raise issues, find solutions and spark-off collective action. The theatrical event merely serves as catalyst, whereby the "entertainment value is interjected with a didactic purpose, but it is a pedagogical method which is collective; it is participatory."[11]

To date, there has not been much research into techniques and mechanisms which characterise that kind of theatre. Publications on the topic are usually concerned with the description of TFD projects in various countries, rather than with an analysis of its theoretical concepts.[12] This study intends to describe structures and techniques inherent in TFD and to demonstrate the interrelationship between the way TFD can be effective and the political and socio-cultural background of the target community. For this purpose, theoretical questions, such as the way in which

8 Cooper, "Who is the Populist?" p. 99.

9 Desai, "Theatre as Praxis," p. 68; for more detailed discussion of popular art forms see Karin Barber, "Popular Arts in Africa," and "Response," *African Studies Review*, Vol. 30, no. 3, September 1987; Mary Jo Arnoldi, "Rethinking Definitions of African Traditional and Popular Arts," *African Studies Review*, Vol. 30, no. 3, September 1987; Donald Cosentino, "Omnes Cultura Tres Partes Divisa Est?" *African Studies Review*, Vol. 30, no. 3, September 1987; Bennetta Jules-Rosette, "Rethinking the Popular Arts in Africa: Problems of Interpretation," *African Studies Review*, Vol. 30, no. 3, September 1987; Frederick Cooper, "Who is the Populist?" *African Studies Review*, Vol. 30, no. 3, September 1987.

10 Ross Kidd, "Popular Theatre and Nonformal Education in the Third World: Five Strands of Experience," in Hansel Ndumbe Eyoh, *Beyond the Theatre* (Bonn: German Foundation for International Development [DSE], 1991), p. 3.

11 Hansel Ndumbe Eyoh, *Beyond the Theatre* (Bonn: German Foundation for International Development [DSE], 1991), p. 3.

12 for a more detailed research report, s. chapter 1.2.

communication works in a specific social setting, and emanating organisational structures will be discussed. Special emphasis will be laid on a sub-category of TFD, as it has emerged in Uganda and other countries during the last three to four years, which I will call Campaign Theatre (CT). CT is a form of TFD which is concerned with raising the consciousness of people on such topics as child care, environmental issues, health care etc. It is increasingly used by GOs, NGOs, and IOs as a part of information campaigns.[13] The notion among the organisations which advocate CT is that with the help of theatre, a message will reach a larger number of people, and also that theatre through its inherent entertainment value is better suited to convey that message than, for instance, a series of lectures. Theatre as a media is chosen because direct interaction between communicators and audience is possible, and developmental processes can be re-emphasized in discussion after the performance.

Uganda has been selected, because due to its political and theatre history, it seems particularly well suited to demonstrate the relationship between TFD and the political and socio-cultural conditions at work. The development of TFD over the last three to four years can be traced back to the country's political situation of the last twenty years and its effect on the theatre as a whole. Two decades of political dictatorship and Civil War did not encourage theatre activities.[14] People were concerned with surviving the turmoil rather than attempting to develop the country. The theatre that survived the twenty years of Civil War was, to a limited extent, political drama, as practised by Robert Serumaga, Nuwa Sentongo, Byron Kawadwa, and, in larger numbers, domestic comedy.[15] Pure comedies, refraining from

---

13 In the following, I will use the terms CT and Theatre for Consciousness raising synonymously; purely project-oriented plays performed to solve a local problem in a community, are not considered in this study.

14 Milton Obote I (1966-1971), Idi Amin (1971-1979), Milton Obote II (1980-1984); s.a. S.R. Karugire, *A Political History of Uganda* (Nairobi, London: Heinemann Educational Books, 1980.); J.J. Jorgensen, *Uganda. A Modern History* (London: Croom Holm, 1981); Nelson Kasfir, *The Shrinking Political Arena. Participation and Ethnicity in African Politics, with a Case Study of Uganda* (Berkeley, Los Angeles, London: University of California Press, 1976); Holger Bernt Hansen and Michael Twaddle, eds., *Uganda Now. Between Decay & Development* (London, Athens, Nairobi: James Currey, Ohio University Press, Heinemann Kenya, 1988); Holger Bernt Hansen and Michael Twaddle, eds., *Changing Uganda* (London, Kampala, Athens, Nairobi: James Currey, Fountain Press, Ohio University Press, Heinemann Kenya, 1991).

15 In my discussion of plays written between 1968 and 1986, I concentrate on works by Robert Serumaga, Nuwa Sentongo, Byron Kawadwa, and Fajil Mandy, because they seem most relevant for describing TFD activities in Uganda today. Other authors

political comment, provided entertainment without endangering the lives of playwrights and actors. Since 1986, however, when the National Resistance Movement (NRM) under President Yoweri Museveni came into power, the situation has changed. Freedom of speech has been re-established, and this development led to a boom in the field of theatre. In the capital, Kampala, alone about 200 theatre groups (non-professional) have been counted; throughout Uganda the number is estimated at 400. New theatre halls that can seat up to 1000 spectators have opened in Kampala, some even in the back-yards of pubs and in school yards. Different types of theatre exist side-by-side: on weekends, many comedies are still performed, but there are also a few plays with political content. Additionally, a new form of theatre has emerged: Theatre for Development (TFD). In the effort to rebuild the country, TFD is becoming increasingly important as a means of information, a fact recognised by the Government which encourages Theatre for Development, and, more recently, by the international aid organisations which, due to the new and free political atmosphere, returned to Uganda to assist in rebuilding the country.

As a result of the unstable political situation over the last two decades, there is a lack of information about theatre in Uganda: there is hardly any critical documentation on theatre productions in the 1980s, and even the works of the literary dramatists of the 1970s have attracted little critical attention. In the first main chapter of this study, I will give an overview of theatre activities between 1968 and 1986, so the evolution of TFD and CT as it is practiced today will be understood. Some plays by the literary dramatists, such as Robert Serumaga, Nuwa Sentongo, Byron Kawadwa and Fajil Mandy, will be discussed in the first part of the chapter. The analysis of their works is important in two respects. First, their influence on TFD as it has developed since 1986 will be demonstrated. Secondly, the relationship between theatre and the political and socio-cultural conditions at work in society will be exemplified when looking at the dramatic techniques developed by Serumaga et al. under the oppressive regimes of Idi Amin and Milton Obote, and comparing them to Theatre for Development as it has emerged after the liberation war had been won by the National Resistance Movement. In the analysis of the plays I will concentrate on the more formal aspects, such as dramatic techniques applied to convey a message to the audience, and on the parallels between those techniques and the

include Jones M.R. Bamwesigye, Elvania Zirimu, Eli N. Kyeyune, Eria Lwanga-Kizza, John Ruganda, Cliff Lubwa p'Chong; for further reference, s. bibliography.

political situation in Uganda at the time. For that purpose, a brief sub-chapter will be included pointing out some of the political events under the regimes of Amin and Obote. The second part of the chapter describes how the theatre scene in Uganda changed when the political atmosphere changed following the takeover by Yoweri Museveni in 1986. With a government devoted to the rebuilding of the war-damaged country, theatre changed from criticising the leadership to supporting it in its efforts of reconstruction. Resultant of that open political climate, TFD started to emerge. Contrary to Theatre for Development projects in other African countries, TFD in Uganda is not applied in order to sensitize the population for a change of the existing political order.[16] Throughout history, popular art forms have been used for purposes of both undermining as well as supporting existing power structures. In Uganda, TFD serves GOs, NGOs and IOs as an instrument to inform and educate Ugandans about development issues. The first TFD activities evolving after 1986 were projects implementing a concrete development aim rather than plays trying to raise awareness. In my description of those projects I concentrate on their structural and organisational side rather than on dramatic techniques applied in the plays. The emphasis being to expose the political and social framework influencing forms of theatre. Besides trying to present the development of Ugandan theatre between 1968 and 1986, the broad survey in the first chapter shows how the phenomenon Campaign Theatre eventually evolved in the specific Ugandan historical and political situation.

The second chapter takes a theoretic approach to CT. In the attempt to analyse Campaign Theatre, its structures and techniques, I soon realised the purely literary/theatrical approach cannot adequately describe it as other complex areas are involved, such as different issues of development politics, health, hygiene, community development et al., and various aspects of communication theory and their application to theatre and development. To fully take into account the phenomenon CT, I combined findings of the different theoretical approaches that seemed relevant. Since CT is employed as a means of mass communication, communication theory as an approach for analysis suggests itself. The questions what kind of arguments occur, what kinds of images and which metaphors are used, and which parts of the audience's consciousness are thus addressed will be explored. Another critical question to pursue is the organisational framework of CT and its influence on the form of the projects. As mentioned, CT is not

16 for a more detailed discussion, s. chapter 2.1.

performed by the target communities, or Ugandans alone. GOs, NGOs and IOs control the productions, which has led to the existence of characteristic organisational structures. Since in CT people belonging to international NGOs as well as Ugandans from different ethnic groups are involved, successful communication must occur between the cultures for the project to be effective. This explains the use of English as the *lingua franca*. Findings of semiotics of culture will therefore be discussed in the theoretical chapter, especially to explain how misunderstandings in intercultural communication occur and can be avoided. Obviously, intercultural communication can only be successful when the participants of the communication process have some knowledge and understanding about each other's cultures. In Uganda, as in other former colonies, we have the situation where Ugandans, through the missionaries and, more recently through Western cultural imports such as TV, news-magazines etc., have some knowledge of social and moral concepts of Europeans whereas the inverse does not hold true. This poses a problem, especially when talking about sensitive topics in health education, such as sexually transmitted diseases (STDs), where a people's sexual habits are involved. I therefore included a sub-chapter discussing the social and moral concepts of Ganda society, since they are essential when judging the effectiveness of a play.[17]

The third major chapter is concerned with the more practical aspects of Campaign Theatre. Initially, issues to be considered when producing a play, such as setting, language, and their influence on the audience's mood will be discussed. The second part of the chapter presents seven CT projects which have been carried out in Uganda between 1989 and 1991. The projects will be described, and methods of performance as well as the content of the plays will be analysed - both in relation to the dramatic techniques developed by the literary playwrights of the sixties and seventies as well as to the theoretical framework discussed in the previous chapter. The plays that I have selected for discussion are all concerned with AIDS. I stress, however, that I focus on this one topic not because Uganda is the only country hit by the disease, but rather because the NRM-Government in its attempt to fight the problem has adopted a very open policy. One unfortunate result of this has been that the AIDS-epidemic in its worst form in many people's perception is now undeservedly linked mainly with Uganda. Upsetting

[17] My description of CT in Uganda mainly focuses on Buganda, the southern region of Uganda which includes the capital, Kampala. This focus is because almost all CT activities are organised in Kampala and taken into the country from there. The organisation of the projects, therefore, is carried out mainly by Baganda.

reports in news-magazines and TV broadcasts come to mind, in which pictures of Ugandan villages are shown where children are the only survivors of the epidemic. In the increasing number of articles and books on the subject, Uganda is usually quoted as the country which is worst hit by the disease. It should be noted, however, that the situation is not confined to Uganda, but also exists in other African countries, especially Zaire, Rwanda, Tanzania, Kenya, Zambia and Zimbabwe - not to speak of Latin-America, Asia, and also Europe. The reason why journalists, scientists, film-directors et al. concentrate so heavily on Uganda has to do with the fact that the Ugandan Government quite unlike those of many other African countries, adopted a very open attitude as far as AIDS information and research are concerned. The Government does not hide the fact that the number of people who are already infected is alarmingly high. Instead, it has been realised that the further spread of the disease must be prevented, and that proper treatment for those already infected has to be provided. Information about infection and prevention must be made available to everybody. There have been, for example, government-sponsored information campaigns which promoted slogans like "love carefully" and "zero grazing."[18] Through its open policy the Government attempts to encourage Ugandan NGOs, self-help groups and artists to join the campaign. It is in accordance with this open policy that, as early as 1986, when the first AIDS cases were discovered, or rather, identified, there were no restrictions placed on foreign researchers and journalists to report and publish what they saw.

True, Uganda is badly affected by the disease, but Uganda is also the country which first among African countries reacted rigorously to the AIDS catastrophe, "both at the level of popular culture and in terms of government intervention."[19] Uganda was the first African country to establish an indigenous self-help group, TASO (The AIDS Support Organisation), which started working as early as 1987. TASO provides counselling for families and patients, and gives work to some of them. As an NGO, it has gained world-wide respect, and many foreign journalists and researchers come to Uganda especially to learn more about its work.

---

[18] The term "zero grazing" is derived from cattle breeding where it refers to cattle being kept on their own property. In the AIDS campaign it is used as a slogan promoting fidelity.

[19] John Ryle, "A Dance of Death," *TLS*, April 27-May 3, 1990, p. 437.

Not only the Government and TASO, but international aid organisations as well are committed to fight AIDS, and they increasingly realise that theatre can be a very effective tool to spread information. Consequently, many plays concerned with the disease were performed between 1989 and 1991, providing a singular example for the phenomenon of CT and its various approaches.

1.2. The Current State of Research

The history of didactic theatre in Africa goes back to the colonial times. The first reports appeared in the 1940s when Margaret Macpherson related about the use of TFD in Uganda.[20] Similar reports exist by A. Dickson and A.K. Pickering about occasions in West Africa when theatre was employed in the service of health education.[21] Outside those few articles, there is hardly any documentation on the use of Theatre for Development prior to 1975. It was in the second half of the 1970s and even more so in the 1980s that theatre was employed increasingly for community development, and that articles and books were written about it. Even now, comparatively little critical material on the subject can be found. From the existing articles and books, two major areas in which theatre is applied reveal themselves, i.e. primary health care and adult education/social change. The majority of critical material consists of case studies describing various projects throughout Africa where theatre has been used.[22] They are concerned with discussing theatrical approaches rather than theoretical or organisational concepts which characterise TFD. The *Laedza Batanani* project in Botswana, the Samaru projects in Nigeria and the Kamiriithu project in Kenya are

---

20 Margaret Macpherson, "Plays and People: an Examination of Three Ugandan Dramatists: Byron Kawadwa, John Ruganda, and Robert Serumaga," in *The Writer and Society in Africa: the Last Fifty Years and Prospects for the Next*, Makerere Golden Jubilee Writers' Workshops, Paper no. 4 (Nairobi, 1972).

21 A. Dickson, "Mass Education in the Gold Coast and Togo-Land," *Mass Education Bulletin*, 1, no. 3, 1950, pp. 50-53; A.K. Pickering, "Village Drama in Ghana," *Fundamental and Adult Education*, no. 4, 1957, pp. 178-183.

22 T. Shank, "The Theatre and Social Change: Principles and Techniques," *Young Cinema and Theatre*, 1, 1977, pp. 3-12; David Kerr, "Didactic Theatre in Africa," *Harvard Educational Review 51*, no. 1, 1981, pp. 145-155; R. Kidd, "Liberation or Domestication: Popular Theatre and Non-Formal Education in Africa," *Young Cinema and Theatre*, no. 4, 1982, pp. 8-17; John Hodgson, "Theatre in Education," *Theatre Quarterly*, Vol. 1, no. 1, January-March 1971, pp. 57-60; R. Tandon, "The Interlinkages between Primary Health Care and Adult Education," *Convergence*, 15, no. 2, 1982, pp. 3-13; Nancy Edwards, "The Role of Drama in Primary Health Care," *Educational Broadcasting International*, 14, no. 2, 1981, pp. 85-89.

doubtlessly the three projects covered most extensively by critics. There exist, for instance, a number of articles by Ross Kidd and Martin Byram, two adult educators who were involved in the organisation of *Laedza Batanani*, in which they describe the project and their use of theatrical techniques developed by the Brazilian theatre practitioner Augusto Boal.[23] Similarly, critical articles dealing with the Samaru street theatre projects in Northern Nigeria discuss the methodology of conversations between theatre practitioners and members of the target community, the production of the play, and the follow-up actions, as they have developed over the years.[24] In a book edited by Harry Hagher on the use of TFD in Nigeria, the development of TFD and methods as applied in the Samaru projects are summarized comprehensively.[25] Similar to the literature discussing *Laedza Batanani* and the Samaru projects, books and articles on the Kamiriithu project in Kenya stress the ideological side rather than theoretical or historical contexts. In their analyses of Kamiriithu, critics focus on the impact of theatre as an instrument for the oppressed people to bring about social change.[26]

Besides the more practical description of case studies, a number of articles have been written on the use of traditional folk media, i.e. theatre,

---

23 R. Kidd. "Liberation or Domestication: Popular Theatre and Non-formal Education in Africa," *Young Cinema and Theatre*, no. 3, 1982, pp. 8-17; R. Kidd and M. Byram, "Demystifying Pseudo-Freirian Development. The Case of Laedza Batanani," *Community Development Journal*, 1712, 1982, pp. 91-105; R. Kidd and M. Byram. "Popular Theatre and Development: a Botswana Case Study," *Convergence*, 10, no. 2, 1977, pp. 20-30; R. Kidd and M. Byram, "Popular Theatre as a Tool for Community Education in Botswana," *Assignment Children: a Journal Concerned with Children, Women and Youth in Development*, (Unicef), no. 44, 1978, pp. 35-65.

24 Ross Kidd, "Plays for Farmers: Popular Drama Workshops in Northern Nigeria. Stage Two: From Outside-in to Inside-out," *Théâtre International*, no. 6, 2, 1982, pp. 25-44; Oga S. Abah, "Popular Theatre as Integration and Conscientation: the example of the Katsina-Ala (Nigeria) Project," *Ifda dossier*, 43, July/August 1985, pp. 3-14; Ahmadu Bello Collective, "Plays for Farmers: Popular Drama Workshops in Northern Nigeria. Stage One: the Ahmadu Bello Initiative," *Théâtre International*, no. 6, 2, 1982, pp. 21-24; M. Crow a. M. Etherton, "Wasan Manoma: Community Theatre in the Soba District of Kaduna State," *Savanna*, Ahmadu Bello University, Zaria, 8, 1979, pp. 6-12;

25 Iyorwuese Harry Hagher, ed., *The Practice of Community Theatre in Nigeria* (Jos: Society of Nigerian Theatre Artists (SONTA), 1991).

26 Penina Muhando Mlama, *Culture and Development. The Popular Theatre Aproach in Africa* (Uppsala: the Scandinavian Institute of African Studies, 1991); Ingrid Björkman, *'Mother Sing for Me.' People's Theatre in Kenya* (London and New Jersey: Zed Books Ltd., 1989); Ngugi wa Mirii, "Literacy for and by the People: Kenya's Kamiriithu Project," *Convergence*, 8, no. 4, 1980, pp. 55-61; et al.

for community development.[27] Those articles have mainly been written in the 1980s when a change of attitude in development politics started to spread, and the search for new media had begun.

The various TFD activities in Africa are best summarized in the books by Kees Epskamp and Penina Muhando Mlama.[28] They both stress the connection between culture, development and communication. Neither, however, goes into the theoretical implications of this relationship.

So far, there has been no research into CT - a form of TFD that has only emerged recently. Existing publications on TFD focus on theatre as it is applied by adult and health educators, or, as in the Kamiriithu project (Kenya), on theatre as an instrument against oppression. Theatre as used by GOs, NGOs and IOs in their information campaigns has heretofore been neglected by the critics. The existing accounts of TFD projects do not consider to full extent the historical, political and social dimensions in which Theatre for Development is embedded. This study tries to do both, i.e. describe the phenomenon CT in the context of one country's - Uganda's - political, cultural, social and historical framework.

---

27 N.J. Colletta, "Folk Culture and Development: Cultural Genocide or Cultural Revitalization?" *Convergence*, 10, no. 2, 1977, pp. 9-19; J.A. Lent, "Grassroots Rennaissance: the Increasing Importance of Folk Media in Third World Nations," *Asian Folklore Studies 39*, no. 2, 1980, pp. 145-162; Dickson M. Mwansa, "Theatre as a Tool for Communication," *Ifda dossier*, no. 42, 1984, pp. 23-32; K.N. Bame, "Comic Plays in Ghana: an Indigenous Art Form for Rural Social Change," *Rural Africana*, 27, 1975, pp. 25-41; G.S. Fehrsen, W. Shaska, B. Simon, "The Use of Traditional Means of Communication in an African Community," *International Journal of Health Education*, 22, no. 2, 1979, pp. 122-124; Gaurav Desai, "Theater as Praxis: Discursive Strategies in African Popular Theater," *African Studies Review*, Vol. 33, no. 1, April 1990, pp. 65-92; Karin Barber, "Popular Arts in Africa," *African Studies Review*, Vol. 30, no. 3, September 1987, pp. 1-78.

28 Kees Epskamp, ed., *Theatre in Search of Social Change* (The Hague: CESO, 1984).

2. THEATRE IN UGANDA

2.1. Popular Theatre - Theatre for Development

In order to have a better understanding of TFD in Uganda, a look at other Theatre for Development activities on the continent is helpful. The political orientation of Theatre for Development in Uganda stands in contrast to the popular theatre movements in most other African countries. Whereas TFD in Uganda serves as a government instrument for change, in countries such as Botswana, Nigeria, Lesotho, Kenya, Zimbabwe et al., it is used by theatre practitioners and adult educators as a media for the people to articulate criticism of the respective governments. A comparison of some of those countries with Uganda shows that the varying political and socio-cultural conditions account for the difference. In her 1991 survey of TFD activities in Africa, Penina Muhando Mlama convincingly establishes a connection between the economic, political and social crises most African countries face and the consolidation of the popular theatre tradition. She draws attention to the fact that the masses in Africa today are more aware than in the 1960s, of the fact that those who are in power are mainly interested in maintaining their power rather than in the welfare of the people. It had become obvious that "the alliance of most of the national ruling classes with international capital to exploit the rest of the people has not helped the situation."[1] In this environment, the usefulness of popular theatre has been realised as a tool in the "struggle against the forces undermining people's welfare."[2] Its goal is to make people aware of the forces which determine their living conditions and to draw them as active participants into the development process by furthering the expression of their own viewpoints and actions to improve their conditions.

Among the countries most actively involved in creating models of Theatre for Development are Malawi, Botswana, Swaziland, Lesotho, Sierra Leone, Nigeria, Cameroon, Zimbabwe, Zambia, Kenya and Tanzania. One of the first projects, the *Laedza Batanani Popular Theatre Programme*, took place in Botswana in 1974. It was an adult education programme which initially lasted one year with weekly events. A team of actors toured the villages, put on performances, and organised discussions. Preceeding the

1 Penina Muhando Mlama, *Culture and Development*, p. 67.

2 ibid., p. 67.

performances, workshops with community representatives were held and priority issues were identified. Local councillors lead the campaign, and extension workers as local organizers of community participation were also involved. Typical topics of the performances of *Laedza Batanani* included cattle theft, inflation, unemployment, the effect of migrant labour on communities and families, conflicts between traditional and modern practices, education and health problems.[3] The significance of *Laedza Batanani* is that it introduced two-way communication into development projects: people were made aware of their situation, encouraged to look at their problems and take action to solve them, instead of merely receiving messages from government employees.

The organizers of *Laedza Batanani* found acceptance of the project among community members so encouraging that the project was extended and continued for several years. The success of *Laedza Batanani* soon influenced similar projects in Swaziland, Lesotho, Zambia, and Malawi.[4] The organizers of the Maratholi Travelling Theatre in Lesotho, however, soon dropped the *Laedza Batanani* approach; it had been realised that the *Laedza Batanani* approach does not make theatre authentically popular in the sense that it is the people's own communication medium.[5] The workshops were instigated by officials and the villagers were not actively involved in the process of analysing the information, scripting the drama and performing the plays. Rather, the extension workers collected information from the villagers, analysed it and worked out a production.

In 1981 the Ahmadou Bello University (ABU) Theatre group in Nigeria initiated an improved approach in one of their rural theatre workshops in the Bomo area. With the Bomo model, they applied Augusto Boal's theatre methodology in order to involve the villagers more than merely as a passive audience. The Brazilian theatre practitioner Boal had developed a technique, the so-called Forum Theatre, where the actors present a problem of the community that needs to be solved. Just before the solution, however, they interrupt the play and ask the audience to suggest possible solutions. The actors encourage spectators to step on stage and present the ending themselves. The ABU theatre group used Boal's Forum

---

3 s.a. M. Byram, 1981, quoted in Mlama, *Culture and Development*, p. 76.

4 for a more detailed discussion s.a. Kidd, 1983; Byram, 1981; in Mlama, *Culture and Development*.

5 s.a. Zakes Mda and Ross Kidd, quoted in Mlama, *Culture and Development*, p. 76.

Theatre so that the audience was actively involved in a critical analysis of what was presented:

> Each scene required village participation: our own team members played the bureaucrats but all the other roles were assigned to the villagers. They took up their roles very easily and added much more depth to the discussion of the issues in the play. For example, in the village co-op meeting scene, one of the villagers spontaneously raised the issue of bribing the government store official (as possible strategy) and another expressed his disgruntlement with the co-op and demanded his membership fee back. Another villager in this meeting accused the co-op representative of "chopping" (misappropriating) the members' money.
>
> At the end of the fertilizer scene we stopped and asked for their reaction. One man said we had not shown how people wait for days in the queue outside the government store. So we replayed the government store scene under his direction, creating a huge line-up (made of the villagers), lots of shoving and jockeying for position within the line, the storekeeper ignoring people in the line and keeping everyone waiting, the trader being challenged by the farmers when he tried to jump the queue, the whole line bursting into the storekeeper's office when they overheard the trader bribing the storekeeper, and the agricultural officer eventually driving the farmers out of the store.[6]

With this approach core actors still come from outside, but members of the community actively discuss issues, present their own point of view by becoming actors themselves and "in the process raising their consciousness and critical awareness of their reality."[7] This is also the approach that characterizes the later works of the Maratholi Travelling Theatre from Lesotho, and to which the group refers as *Theatre for Conscientization*. It was again adopted in Malawi in 1986 by the Liwonde Primary Health Care Unit together with the Chancellor College Fine and Performing Arts Department, when a Public Health Care project in rural areas was supposed to be implemented.[8] The approach turned out to be quite successful. As a result of the project, the village health committees have protected over forty shallow wells, and 51% of the households have constructed pit latrines as compared to 10% a year earlier. The organizers noted the awareness of general health practices was higher than before the programme.[9]

---

6 Kidd, 1983, quoted in Mlama, *Culture and Development*, p. 78.

7 Mlama, *Culture and Development*, p. 78.

8 ibid., p. 79.

9 ibid., p. 80.

Another workshop on Theatre for Development was held in 1983 in Murewa, Zimbabwe. It was aimed at training theatre workers and developing cadres and local villagers in the skills and methods of a consciousness-raising theatre. The workshop was based on the Ahmadou Bello University model, using Augusto Boal's techniques. It turned out particularly successful owing to an active, deeply-rooted artistic tradition in Zimbabwean popular culture which ensured maximum participation of the community members. As Mlama points out, however, even though the workshop caused quite a stir in the area during its run, it did not have a lasting impact on the use of TFD in Zimbabwe. Nevertheless, the workshop is significant nevertheless, because it showed use of people's own art forms ensures the most effective participation from the community. In previous popular theatre projects the element of drama was over-emphasised and neglected other art forms such as dance and music. A reason for the apparent stress of narrative elements of drama, according to Mlama, is because the projects were largely organized by European expatriates, including people like Ross Kidd, Martin Byram, Andrew Horn, David Kerr, Brian Crow, and Michael Etherton, who, due to their own cultural background, focussed rather exclusively on drama. As other possible reasons she sees either neo-colonial attitudes, "whereby the expatriates deliberately ignored the indigenous theatre forms because they believed in the superiority of European theatrical forms";[10] or simply an insufficient knowledge of theatrical techniques on the side of the organizers. Since most of those expatriates were involved in adult education or the teaching of English literature, their theatrical skills were limited.

One of the most widely known popular theatre events, the Kamiriithu project in Kenya, involved only Kenyans. In 1977 a group of lecturers from the University of Nairobi decided to participate in reviving the Kamiriithu Community Education and Cultural Centre. The first activity was the organization of adult education classes, and the objective of the group was to make those classes a liberating process through which the peasants' awareness of exploitation could be raised. The lecturers, who functioned as facilitators, tried to expose the fact that the poverty in Kamiriithu was caused by an unjust economic system in which a few members of society were exploiting the majority. The participants were encouraged to question the status quo and to see the reasons for their landlessness and poverty. They also became organizers of their own programme by making decisions

10 Mlama, *Culture and Development*, p. 85/6.

on the curriculum, recruiting teachers, and mobilising village support. Looking for a medium that would increase the villagers' participation, the lecturers came up with the concept of popular theatre.[11] Before a play was created, a cultural committee held several meetings to decide on its content. Then, Ngugi wa Thiong'o and Ngugi wa Mirii were asked to draft a play in Kikuyu. The draft was later discussed by the participants, and amendments were made. As a result, the play *Ngahika Ndeenda* (*I will Marry When I Want*) was produced.[12] It tells of a poor farmer who is cheated out of his land by a multinational company which plans to build a factory on the land, in cooperation with a bank and members of the indigenous upper class. Eventually, the farmers and workers realise that they are being exploited, and "a powerful appeal for a unanimous rebellion against exploitation brings down the curtain."[13] Mlama reports there were seven weeks of public rehearsals which culminated in performances that attracted audiences even from outside Kamiriithu.[14] As she points out, the success of the play was due to its ability to encourage the participation of all age groups in the community. The numerous songs, dances and traditional ceremonies contained in the play allowed "the peasants to unleash their rich artistic talents in an expression of their suffering."[15] They felt that the story of their lives, hopes and struggles was told. The performance of *I Will Marry When I Want* was an important event since this was the first time a play had been performed in an indigenous language in Kenya. The production was staged in an open-air theatre that was constructed by the people of Kamiriithu themselves and had room for about 2000 spectators. In 1982, the theatre was razed by the government and the Kamiriithu centre was closed. One of its leading figures, Ngugi wa Thiong'o, was imprisoned between 1977 and 1980, and several other lecturers had to flee Kenya. Today, the Kamiriithu project is seen by many people as "the most successful use of people's theatre in developing critical consciousness and mobilising people for

---

11 ibid., p. 92.

12 ibid., p. 92 .

13 Ingrid Björkman. *'Mother Sing For Me.' People's Theatre in Kenya* (London and New Jersey: Zed books Ltd., 1989), p. 1.

14 Ngugi wa Thiong'o, "Women in Cultural Work: the Fate of Kamiriithu People's Theatre in Kenya," *Development and Dialogue*, Vol. 1-2 (Uppsala: The Dag Hammars-Kjölk, 1982).

15 Mlama, *Culture and Development*, p. 93.

collective action."[16] The reaction reveals that government is well aware of the power of theatre in raising consciousness. As Ingrid Björkman remarks, Ngugi wa Thiongo's three latest novels in Swahili and Kikuyu carry a message similar to that of the play. The novels are freely available in Kenya even though novel-reading is an activity enjoyed by all social classes, and the books in fact reach a large audience, so a ban would not have been unexpected. The real danger, therefore, is perceived not so much in the message or the size of the audience but rather in the fact of performance. The production of *I Will Marry When I Want* posed a threat to the government, because it was not an isolated event; it developed out of a larger cultural enterprise and as such "formed a part of much larger communal efforts attempting to change the image of the rural village of Kamiriithu."[17] It was supposed to instill a sense of dignity, identity and self-respect in the people, thus enabling them to improve their own situation.

This look at various TFD projects in Africa demonstrates the obvious difference to Theatre for Development in Uganda. A brief digression to the country's political history of the last two decades will explain the focus on developmental topics as well as the patterns and techniques we see in Ugandan TFD today.

Under the oppressive regimes of Milton Obote (1966-1971 & 1980-1985) and Idi Amin (1971-1979) artists who commented critically on the political situation risked their lives.[18] A few playwrights nevertheless continued to write plays in which they criticised political events. Attempts of this kind were few and far between and eventually stopped altogether; especially after the killing of Byron Kawadwa, the director of the National Theatre, by Amin's security police, presumably because of his play *St. Lwanga,* and after Robert Serumaga fled into exile. The genre of drama which survived was comedy dealing with social and domestic problems. By focussing on those topics the artists knew they would keep out of trouble. Moreover, comedies were extremely popular with the spectators who in the theatre could forget the terrorism they were subjected to in their daily lives - even if it was only for a few hours.

When in 1986 the National Resistance Movement under Yoweri Museveni came into power, the political situation changed. For the first

---

16 Kidd, 1983, in Mlama, *Culture and Development*.

17 Björkman, *'Mother Sing For Me,'* p. 94.

18 for a more detailed discription of the Obote and Amin regimes, s. chapter 2.2.1.

time in many years, the country experienced a disciplined army which did not rape, loot and kill; thus the security situation for most Ugandans improved.[19] Theatrical activities developed according to the new political atmosphere. Many of the critical artists who had left the country under Amin and Obote have established new lives for themselves in their respective countries of exile and are reluctant to return to Uganda. Consequently, with few exceptions, there is virtually no political drama.[20] Moreover, playwrights still are cautious. After 20 years of oppression and terror, it takes more than a few years to trust a Government's assurance of tolerance and freedom of expression.

What this means is that the majority of plays performed today are still comedies, as during the years of the Obote and Amin regimes. In fact, they are more popular than ever. In a country where few people have access to television, there is a high demand for other forms of entertainment. Theatrical comedies address the social problems most people in post-civil war Uganda face. They are performed in theatre halls as well as in bars, schools, and back-yards. The play *The Prodigal Son* by the Bamazinga Players (1989) is typical. It was performed on weekends in the back-yard of a bar. Its plot is simple and characteristic for popular literature in the third world: a young man comes to town to make his fortune and fails. This theme has also dominated western literature during the period of urbanization and the beginnings of industrialization. Village scenes in which the young man's fate is discussed and commented on alternate with scenes in the city where his 'adventures' with prostitutes and criminals are acted out. In the end, the young man's mother bribes a corrupt policeman to release her son from prison and takes him back to the village.[21] The presentation of city-life is so

---

19 This is mainly true of the south and south-west. There is still rebel activity in the northern part of Uganda. Between 1986 and 1992, many people in the north and north-east were put into camps, their huts were burned down. In those camps, many of them died from hunger, disease and torture. Between 200 000 and 500 000 people were kept in camps. The NRA is held responsible for those horrors. Besides, there are reports that the NRM began to persecute opposition groups (UPA; Uganda National Democratic Army - UNDA; United Democratic Christian Army - UDCA, Uganda People Democracy - UPD; National Army for Liberation of Uganda - NALU) as rebels; and the claims for freedom of expression have to be treated with caution, since there are reports that journalists still get arrested. (s. *Kranich*, no. 7, May 1992, p. 17).

20 Recently, a few plays were performed that openly criticised present political issues. The two most outstanding productions in this respect were *Wounds of Africa* and *30 Years of Bananas*, both by playwright and actor Alex Mukulu.

21 Eckhard Breitinger, "Den Fortschritt inszenieren: Theaterarbeit in der Entwicklungspolitik," *Spektrum*, no. 1, (Universität Bayreuth, Feb. 1990), pp. 37-42.

general that every spectator can see his/her own experiences and problems reflected. Besides giving the audience the feeling that their life is being depicted on stage, comedies, with their slap-stick effects and jokes about soldiers and politicians, also offer a chance to ridicule the very forces of oppression. Characteristically these comedies integrate various elements which most likely account for their popularity: they mix elements of religious morality plays with those of social comedy. The fact they last up to four hours and repeat the same jokes with only slight variations meets the audience's preference for discussion and dialogue, as Breitinger remarks.[22] Moreover, they make it possible to speak about soldiers and politicians publicly: they can be "brought onto the stage as laughing stock after so many years of oppression."[23] The likelihood that comedies, with their realistic depiction of everyday problems, may lead to a more critical awareness and self-analysis of the spectators' own situation should not be underestimated. All those factors taken together account for the fact that shows performed on weekends in pubs or the large theatres which seat 700 to 1000 spectators, are usually sold out.[24]

Since the 1986 change in government theatre has been used as an instrument for development in accordance with a Government's policy of reconstruction. The return to peace after twenty years of unrest, limited the motivation to write plays criticising the new regime. On the contrary, the people, including artists, wanted to make a collective effort to rebuild the social infrastructure. TFD in Uganda has to be seen within the context of government's appeal for help in rebuilding the country.

The connection between theatre and the political and socio-cultural framework within which it takes place becomes evident when comparing topics and techniques applied in the political plays of the 1960s and 70s with those used in Theatre for Development today. To communicate messages to their audiences, all playwrights appeal to the audience's sense of tradition by incorporating folk-elements in their productions; we frequently find folksongs, folkdance and references to legends or proverbs as a strategy to convince the audience. Besides the general attempt to appeal to the spectators' common identity as Ugandans, however, a basic difference in the

---

22 ibid., p. 40.

23 Eckhard Breitinger, "Popular Urban Theatre in Uganda: Between Self-Help and Self-Enrichment," *New Theatre Quarterly*, Vol. VIII, no. 31, August 1992, p. 281.

24 for a detailed discussion, s. Breitinger, "Popular Urban Theatre."

use of folk-material can be discerned. Political playwrights like Serumaga, Sentongo, and others used it to disguise their message, since direct criticism under Obote and Amin was not possible. Today, with an open political atmosphere, it is no longer necessary to hide meaning. TFD artists adapted those same techniques to communicate more clearly to their audiences. A look at Uganda's theatre history of the last twenty years will explain the evolution of Theatre for Development as practised today.

2.2. Theatre between 1968 and 1986

2.2.1. Political background

To show the evolution of the political plays between 1968 and 1986 to the emergence of theatre used in nationwide campaigns for health education (CT), plays by selected political playwrights will be examined in subsequent chapters. Before doing that, however, I want to reiterate the most crucial political events of the years between independence and 1986. The successive terror regimes of Obote I, Amin, and Obote II influenced theatre activities to a considerabale degree, and playwrights such as Serumaga, Sentongo, Kawadwa and Mandy can only be adequately appreciated in light of the political background. In my account, I focus on those salient points that are relevant for the analyses of plays selected for discussion.

Uganda gained independence from the British in 1962. The country had been given a democratic constitution, and the Baganda King, called the Kabaka, was supported by the British as president. Milton Obote, member of the Uganda People's Congress (UPC), became Prime Minister. In 1966, Obote assumed power: after his return from a tour of northern districts, he crushed opposition coming from the right wing of his own party. At a cabinet meeting on 22 February 1966, he arrested the right wing ministers of his cabinet, suspended the 1962 constitution and assumed all state power:

> And then to demonstrate his commitment to parliamentary democracy..., Obote summoned his considerably apprehensive Parliament... "as from this moment the constitution which we had from 9th October 1962 is hereby abrogated (and the blessed Honourables cheered)... NOW THEREFORE WE, the people of Uganda... do resolve... and it is hereby abolished accordingly and the constitution now before us be adopted and is hereby

adopted this day of 15th April 1966... fairly soon you will find your copies in your pigeon holes."[25]

In April 1966, Obote presented an interim constitution to the National Assembly without debate: "the slogan of the new order was 'one country, one Parliament, one Government, one people,' led by an executive President: Milton Obote."[26] After protests from the Kabaka of Buganda, demanding the central government's withdrawal from Buganda, the Kabaka's palace at Lubiri was taken over by Obote's army, and a state of emergency was proclaimed in the area. Buganda was divided into four administrative districts. A year later, in 1967, a new republican constitution was introduced abolishing all traditional rulers and all local legislatures.[27]

Obote's party, the Uganda People's Congress, tried to appear as a party of the masses, "the common man." One of its often-heard slogans was "fighting ignorance, disease, and poverty."[28] The socialist character of Obote's policy was much debated in Uganda at the time. His involvement in the second Congo crisis, where he supported the rebels, and visits to Yugoslavia, China and the Soviet Union in July 1966 gave rise to the speculation that the regime was "moving to increased state control of the economy and a left-of-centre foreign policy."[29] As Sathyamurthy points out, however, Obote's main ideological commitment was to nationalism. He merely used socialist rhetoric in his desire to ensure the consolidation of Uganda's national unity: his "commitment to bringing about a fairer distribution of the wealth produced by Ugandan labour began to falter almost immediately after the well-known *pronuncimientos* of 1970 (especially the Nakivubo announcements) were issued."[30]

Due to a lack of support in his own party, to increasing dependence on the army, to a failed agricultural reform and a spreading discontent with his autoritarian leadership, Obote's position weakened. In 1971, Sergeant Idi Amin assumed power through a military coup. Amin's military dictatorship

---

25 S.R. Karugire, *The Roots of Instability in Uganda* (Kampala: The New Vision printing and Publishing Co-operation, 1988), p. 234.

26 Jan Jelmert Jorgensen, *Uganda. A Modern History* (London: Croom Helm, 1981), p. 230.

27 ibid., p. 231.

28 ibid, p. 214.

29 ibid, p. 229.

30 T.V. Sathyamurthy, *The Political Development of Uganda: 1900-1986* (Hants, England: Gower, 1986), p. 467.

brought worldwide attention to Uganda for several reasons. First, in 1972, Amin expelled approximately 50 000 Asians, mainly Indians, from the country. The Asians had been engaged in trade and small scale industries, and their expulsion enabled members of the bureaucracy to enrich themselves by usurping the Asian property. Secondly, because of the terrorism the population was subjected to under Amin's terror regime. The brutal excesses of his regime caused the death of about 200 000 Ugandans - the exact number is not known. Although more people than just Idi Amin were involved in the brutal mass killings, it was the person Amin who was the focus of world wide attention, the political clowneries of the publicity-addicted Idi Amin - in his narrow-mindedness and brutality a typical product of colonial armies ("die schlagzeilenträchtigen politischen Clownerien des publizitätssüchtigen Amin - in seiner Beschränktheit und Brutalität ein typisches Produkt kolonialer Armeen").[31] Not only the colonial history made Amin what he was; his childhood set the tone for his reliance on witchcraft and witch doctors. His mother was a Lugbara, "known to be steeped in witchcraft."[32] She left Amin's father when Amin was still a baby and went to Lugazi to live among other Lugbaras who were working the sugar-cane estates of rich Asian families. As a witch, she then moved on to the outskirts of the barracks of the King's African rifles at a place called Buikwe.[33] She went to live with Corporal Yafesi Yasin, a clerk in 'D' Company of the 4th King's African Rifles, and that brought her into Jinja barracks. George Ivan Smith draws the conclusion that due to the rootless, restless childhood of Idi Amin, it is not surprising he took up images and knowledge of a "Sorcerer's Apprentice."[34] His obsession with witchcraft was also confirmed by Henry Kyemba, his former Health minister, who fled the country in 1977. Kyemba reports on one occasion in September 1976, when they were talking at the President's Lodge in Nakasero, Amin said: "I have eaten human meat. It is very salty, even more salty than leopard meat." In his book,[35] Kyemba writes of Amin's belief in witchcraft: "He regularly visits witch doctors both in Jinja (...) and in Kampala... Amin usually goes to them because he needs advice on some problem or other - he may wish to have an

---

31 *Kranich. Uganda Nachrichten*, no. 1, no year, p. 7.

32 George Ivan Smith, *Ghosts of Kampala* (London: Weidenfeld and Nicolson, 1980), p. 42.

33 ibid, p. 43.

34 ibid, p. 43.

35 Henry Kyemba, *State of Blood* (USA, and Corgi, UK: Paddington Press).

'enemy' name, for instance, or he may want to know what action to take to avoid assassination...."[36] One house servant, who later fled to Kenya, even claims that Amin kept severed heads and human organs in the refrigerator of one of his homes.[37] The servant was working in one of the presidential residences in Kampala when Amin's fifth wife, Sarah, discovered the head of her former lover in the refrigerator.

The extended account of Amin's belief in sorcery is given, because it plays a crucial role in one of the plays which will be discussed later.[38] I do not mean to imply that only Idi Amin was responsible for the brutal killings under his regime. As Semakula Kiwanuka remarks, Amin's record of murder was not the work of one man. Members of all parts of society, from different ethnic, religious and professional groups were involved in the dealings of the notorious secret service, the State Research Bureau: "Numerous professional men and women, top men in the university, in the corporations, in the civil service, in medicine plus nearly all the Medical Superintendents were members of the dreaded State Research Bureau."[39] As the brutalities and corruption within the Amin regime increased, so did the intelligence network. In every locality, Government bodies were spying on each other. Smith reports that by 1977 and 1978, when training schemes had increased the number of agents, their greed for money caused the loss of many innocent lives: "Because they had learnt to live in a realm dependent upon material gains, the agents began arresting any Ugandans who had the slightest appearance of affluence. They could take them to prison without stating any known offence. They found means by which they could obtain signatures from the captive to get funds from his family or from his bank - and then, when the money ran out, the captive died."[40]

In 1979 Idi Amin was driven from power by the Tanzanian army, but in the aftermath the two short successive governments under Yusuf Lule and Godfrey Binaisa plunged the country even deeper into political and economic chaos. Eventually, in maniplulated elections held in 1980, Obote came back into power again. Despite the obvious manipulation of the

---

36 in Dan Wooding and Ray Barnett, *Uganda Holocaust* (Grand Rapids, Michigan: Zondervan Publishing House, 1980), p. 69.

37 ibid., p. 69/70.

38 s. chapter 2.2.2. Nuwa Sentongo, *The Invisible Bond*.

39 Semakula Kiwanuka, *Amin and the Tragedy of Uganda* (München, London: Weltforum Verlag, 1979), p. 195.

40 Smith, *Ghosts of Kampala*, p. 126.

elections, they were recognised by an international team of observers from Commonwealth States. Obote's second regime, which lasted until 1985, did not bring the hoped for peace and stability to Uganda. Under the pretext of fighting guerilla groups, "the soldiers of the Ugandan army have engaged in an orgy of killing, rape and looting, especially but not only in the thickly populated villages of Buganda districts."[41] Estimates speak of 400 000 deaths in the Luwero district alone.

Yoweri Museveni, together with the National Resistance Army (NRA), who had been fighting against the Obote regime since 1981, profited from the increasingly bad security situation in the country. Because of their considerate and disciplined behaviour towards the population, the soldiers of the NRA enjoyed the confidence and support of the farmers who were subjected to the constant attacks of the Government army. In 1986, Yoweri Museveni won the liberation war and is now the President of Uganda.

2.2.2. Robert Serumaga

In 1968, after Obote abolished the monarchies in Uganda,[42] it became clear that direct political comments in theatre plays or literature could become dangerous for the artists.[43] During that year, the writer Wycliff Kyingi made a comment about Obote's usurpation of power in his Luganda radio serial, *Wokulira*. The transmission of the episode happened to coincide with the day on which Obote came into power. The show was banned immediately, and the cast was put into prison. After that Ugandan artists realised if they wanted to comment on the political situation in their country, they had to find alternative forms which would camouflage the political messages of the play. Authors developed methods of using folk-material which besides allowing indirect political comments, also served the purpose of appealing to the emotions of the audience. Among the playwrights who worked during that period, especially Robert Serumaga presents a dynamic approach to folklore. Where they are used in TFD plays, the techniques he applied have survived to the present day.

---

41 Sathyamurthy, *The Political Development of Uganda*, p. 671.

42 Until 1968, the south and south-west of Uganda was ruled by four Kingdoms: Buganda, Toro, Ankole, and Bunyoro.

43 Rose Mbowa, "Ugandan Literature," Ringvorlesung, Bayreuth University, 11 July 1991, unpublished.

Serumaga first became involved in theatre in Dublin, Ireland, as an undergraduate student, and later in London as a radio producer. Andrew Horn regards Serumaga's work with such theatre forms as variety and revue in U.K. as seminal for his later works; a stand-up comic in theatre is a solitary and isolated person unsupported by other actors or elaborate stageing. This isolation is a central characteristic of major characters in Serumaga's plays, "for each of his main characters is a solo-showman, and each of the plots pivots on this single self-dramatizing figure - one deeply defined introspective consciousness - around whom other, flatter characters are used merely as foils."[44] Four of Serumaga's plays will be analysed as they are relevant for a discussion of present day TFD for two reasons. First, the use of dramatic techniques developed by the author over the years is of interest. His experiments with folk material to convey his message to the audience but at the same time hide the political criticism from the leaders clearly shows the relationship between theatre and the political context in which it takes place, especially when compared to the dramatic techniques applied in TFD under a democratic Government.[45] Second, by opposing the interpretations of critics belonging to two different cultures, i.e. the American Andrew Horn and the Ugandan Rose Mbowa, this relationship will be revealed on another level. The difference between the interpretations points to the fact that a play can only be understood with a thorough knowledge of the political, social and historical situation of a country. Obviously, this also applies to the production of plays, as we shall see in more detail when discussing TFD.

2.2.1.1. *A Play* (1967)

Serumaga's first play, *A Play*, was staged at the National Theatre in Kampala in October 1967 and was performed without act, scene or interval divisions. Horn points out that it was written for a conventional box set, proscenium arch and a naturalistic setting, with an expressionist dream-scene.[46] *A Play* is still realistic, with only the dream-scene hinting at the author's abandoning of realistic stage conventions in his later works: in his second play, *Majangwa* he used absurdist elements, and in *Renga Moi*

44 Andrew Horn, "Individualism and Community in the Theatre of Serumaga." in *African Literature Today 12: New Writing, New Approaches*. ed. Eldred Durosimi Jones and Eustace Palmer (London, Ibadan, Nairobi: Heinemann, 1982), p. 24.

45 s. discussion of the case studies in chapter 4.

46 Horn, "Individualism and Community," p. 24.

African ritual and elements of Grotowski's theatre. The action takes place on the evening of the protagonist's, Mutimukulu, wedding anniversary with his wife, Rose; it is also the evening Rose died. Mutimukulu is alone in the house until two tramps, an Old Man and a Young Man, join him. Before they appear, Mutimukulu has had a dream in which the Head of the god Mukasa, the benign Kiganda god of Thunder, appears and demands Mutimukulu to tell the truth. Mukasa speaks of guilt that has to be revealed, and of lies:

> Mutimukulu, what have you done?...
> I am Mukasa, God of thunder and lighting.
> I am crime-is-dry-meat-that-never-rots.
> I am poison, which once eaten will show up sometime.
> Death holds no secrets for me, and I dig guilt out
> of the darkness of men's souls.
> There is an anthill where I am sitting,
> And you and the truth have parted, and gone your different ways.
> When you meet on the other side of the raise ground,
> The truth will have become a leopard with horns on its head.
> Will you let it eat you, or will you speak out in its face?[47]

During the play, it remains unclear what Mutimukulu is guilty of. His wife Rose seems to have been shot by her two lovers, John and Peter, who wanted to kill Mutimukulu in a chieftaincy struggle. In the dream scene, they come to Mutimukulu's house claiming that Rose had invited them to her wedding anniversary. They declare Mutimukulu mad when he informs them that Rose is dead. When Rose eventually enters the house, Mutimukulu forces John and Peter to shoot her again; since she is already dead she cannot be killed a second time. When Rose is shot again, her relatives come to take revenge on the killers. They kill John and Peter, and the two tramps leave just before the mob attacks Mutimukulu. At that point, the housegirl comes in and awakens him, whereupon he realises he has been dreaming. The play ends with the rather mysterious appearance of a doctor who actually is the Old Man.

In *A Play*, Serumaga explores the existential anguish of the isolated individual, against whom even forces such as the benign, healing god, Mukasa, are turned. It "seems to hover between an exposition of nihilism - life as pointless 'play' between birth and death...."[48] The atmosphere is

---

47 Robert Serumaga, *Majangwa and A Play* (Nairobi: East African Publishing House, 1974), p. 57.

48 Horn, "Individualism and Community," p. 26.

reminiscent of Samuel Beckett's *Waiting For Godot*,[49] the two characters Peter and John strongly resembling Vladimir and Estragon. Like Vladimir and Estragon, most of Peter's and John's time on stage is spent at play, which is also the reason for the title, *A Play*: the game of the wife's re-murder,[50] the game of Heavensgate,[51] and the game of the hanging.[52]

In addition to discussing problems of the individual in general, Serumaga also comments on the political situation in Uganda. When trying to understand *A Play*, one must remember that Serumaga was a royalist. When he returned from Dublin, he was disillusioned by Obote's abolition of the Kingdoms and wanted to express that disillusionment through the highly symbolic characters in *A Play* exploring how the individual had been involved in the destruction of the monarchy that seemingly had such strong roots in Baganda society.[53] Mutimukulu can be seen as an aspect of the self, together with the Old Man and the Young Man: "the three of us - a lifetime." Together, they symbolize the individual life. Rose symbolises the Kingdom of Buganda. She is killed like that Kingdom which to many seemed as beautiful as a rose. That destruction is re-enacted when Mutimukulu forces John and Peter to kill Rose again. The frequent references by Mutimukulu to the time when his wife died, "Five years ago, my wife died," function as hints to the audience about the real significance of *A Play*. In Mutimukulu's dream, the role of the individual in the destruction of the monarchy is being explored. Questions as to what is truth, what has happened, who destroyed the Kingdom, are raised. The involvement of Bugandan society in its destruction is suggested through the killing of Rose by John and Peter.[54]

Rose Mbowa convincingly interpretes the re-appearance of the Old Man as doctor at the end of the play as a representation of the future.

---

49 To stress the parallels between *A Play* and Beckett's play *Waiting For Godot*, Horn points to two quotations from *Waiting For Godot*: Pozzo: "They give birth astride of a grave, the light gleams an instant, then it's night once more" (p. 89); and Vladimir: "Astride of a grave and a difficult birth. Down in the hole, lingeringly, the grave-digger puts on the forceps. We have time to grow old. The air is full of our cries" (p. 90-1).

50 *A Play*, p. 80-2.

51 ibid., p. 93-4.

52 ibid., p. 95; s.a. Horn, "Individualism and Community."

53 Mbowa, "Ugandan Literature." Mbowa was a member of the cast in the 1977 production at the National Theatre.

54 ibid.

Mutimukulu would have become like the Old Man had his past been different. In his past, which is represented by the Young Man, he lived a careless life without thinking, which may be the reason for his, as she sees it, mental sickness.[55] Andrew Horn, on the other hand, regards the play's end as a flaw: "His use of a single actor to play both the Old Man and the Doctor (...) serves only to diminish the quality of indeterminate reality which Serumaga has laboured so hard to establish, suggesting that the play's action has been only a lunatic hallucination, a *rève á clef*, reducing Mutimukulu's existential anguish to a clinical curiosity." [56]

The differences in the assessments of the ending exemplify the different points of view on which these interpretations are based. Rose Mbowa interprets Serumaga's play from a Ugandan viewpoint as a disguised comment on the political situation at the time. Andrew Horn puts the play in a wider context, stressing the dilemma of the individual in a Western way, without drawing the connections to the specific Ugandan situation. The same varying viewpoints as in *A Play* appear again when looking at Horn's and Mbowa's interpretations of Serumaga's next play, *Majangwa*.

2.2.1.2. *Majangwa* (1971)

Majangwa is considered a "far more adventurous work" by Horn, because the personal illusions are "more purposefully shaped and the eponymous central character more richly realised."[57] Mbowa relates that in *Majangwa* Serumaga tried once more to communicate his political views to the audience through a form that would not give away the message explicitly. She tells that during the performance of *A Play*, the actors on stage expected to be arrested any minute. Nothing happened, however, because the play was so complicated that it was not understood. Consequently, Serumaga adopted another strategy in *Majangwa*.

Majangwa was a real person: a traditional drummer, he would walk the streets and market areas in and around Kampala, earning his living playing the drum. His wife, Nakirijja, would accompany him and dance. Society, however, demanded more entertainment, and eventually, Majangwa and his wife started kissing in public, and then progressed to having sex on the

55 ibid.

56 Horn, "Individualism and Community," p. 27.

57 ibid., p. 32.

pavement, so that the people would get aroused and throw money at them. As with *A Play*, Horn's and Mbowa's interpretations of *Majangwa* differ. Andrew Horn interprets *Majangwa* as a "reflection on the realities of the artist's role in society,"[58] with Majangwa himself standing in the tradition of the romantic artist, whereas Rose Mbowa sees it as a comment on the sickness of society in Amin's time. Horn's viewpoint of *Majangwa*, while accurate, again lacks the Ugandan component. The play was written and performed in Kampala during Amin's dictatorship, and there are clear parallels to actual events of that time, which should not be ignored.

The play opens with Majangwa and Nakirijja walking on a road. Looking for a place to spend the night, Majangwa begins to reflect about his life. It is Nakirijja, however, bitter and unnerved by years of self-degradation and humiliation, who recalls what really has happened in their lives: how they have been compelled first to vary their performances to include public kissing, and eventually a display of copulation. Majangwa states, that this had not just been a public display of sex for a market audience, but rather a chance for renewal and regeneration of the audience, "a ritualistic act of sympathetic healing":[59]

> Did you think we were cheap entertainers? No, woman, I see it all now. We were the gods' go-betweeners, putting bones back into broken limbs. Yes, five shillings and they watched us, and waited and hoped that a whiff of passion would rub off on them and arouse them. The chance of a cure, woman, that's what we were to them.[60]

It seems that by transferring their vitality to the audience, Majangwa and Nakirijja themselves have become barren and impotent:

Nakirijja:	Do you think we will ever have a child? (silence)
Majangwa:	(very sadly) I don't know.
Nakirijja:	My womb has been silent for too long.
Majangwa:	It may not be your fault.
Nakirijja:	... I wanted a child so much...
Majangwa:	Oh, I don't know, woman. I have drunk from the earthen bowl many times, taken to the root and examined the cock's entrails, but nothing seems to add any edge to my approach. What else can I do but wait?[61]

---

58 ibid., p. 32.

59 ibid., p. 32

60 *Majangwa*, p. 21.

61 ibid., p. 19.

Although Majangwa and Nakirijja forgo having children in order to regenerate society, their sacrifice is not appreciated. Their house was burnt down, with all their belongings, and, most important, their drum.

Majangwa and Nakirijja now see a chance to regenerate themselves. In the forest clearing, they watch for people making love on the back seats of their cars having stopped on their way home from the cinemas. By watching them having sex, just as the people in the markets watched Majangwa and Nakirijja having sex on the pavement, they hope they will have a chance for rejuvenation. While waiting for the lovers they fall asleep. Majangwa has a dream in which Death appears to him in a mime scene. The forest clearing they have choosen for their regeneration happens to be at Tanda where, according to legend, death descended into the earth, and from where he emerges to claim the living.[62]

Majangwa and Nakirijja represent a Uganda whose society is sick and in need of rejuvenation. There is little hope, however, to achieve this as death is all around. At the end, when a car finally arrives, it is not the lovers that Majangwa and Nakirijja are waiting for, but someone throwing a body from the car. Rose Mbowa, who worked with Serumaga at Makerere University, relates that while Serumaga was still writing the play, Amin had a business tycoon, Michael Kaggwa, killed and burned in his Mercedes Benz. Serumaga wrote the ending of the play after hearing of this incident. The final scene is a clear comment on Uganda: people are waiting in hope, but there is only death.[63]

I think, when discussing *Majangwa,* its specific relation to Ugandan politics of the time should not be marginalized. While Horn's interpretation

---

62 In the legend, Kintu lives alone on earth. One day, Gulu (God) steals Kintu's cow and takes it to Heaven. Kintu follows and has to fulfill several tasks in order to regain his cow. After successfully carrying out the tasks, Kintu sees Nambi, Gulu's daughter, and falls in love with her. With Gulu's consent, he takes her back to earth as his wife. Before they leave, Gulu admonishes them to go immediately and not look back so that Nambi's brother Walumbe, symbolizing death, will never find them. On their way down to earth, however, Nambi discovers that she has forgotten the millet for her hen. Despite Kintu's apprehensions she goes back to Heaven to collect it. Walumbe sees her and follows her and Kintu to earth, where he haunts them and their children. They get help from Nambi's other brother, Kaikuzi, who is sent by Gulu to take Walumbe back to Heaven. Walumbe flees from Kaikuzi into a hole below the earth, but eventually manages to free himself, because Nambi's and Kintu's children did not obey Kaikuzi's orders to stay quietly in their house, thus making Walumbe's escape possible. From then on, death existed on earth and kept emerging from the hole in the ground to claim the living.

63 Mbowa, "Ugandan Literature"

of *Majangwa* as exploring the artist's role in society is doubtlessly true, it is too narrowly focussed. The parallel between the ending of *Majangwa* and the murder of Michael Kaggwa is made obvious when Majangwa, before running away with Nakirijja, suggests that they burn the body so there would be no evidence and they would not be accused of murder.

In *Majangwa*, Serumaga communicates his message more clearly than in *A Play*. He uses traditional material like the legend of Kintu, and the life of Majangwa, a public figure of the 1950s familiar to many Ugandans, to complement the allusions to topical events. By referring to that common cultural and political knowledge, the author disguises the political content and thus leaves room for interpretations like Horn's, but at the same time the political message is understood by any Ugandan audience familiar with the events of the time. Clearly, Serumaga was looking for devices that would communicate better to the audience. The concentration on narrative folk-elements, like myths and legends, however, poses a danger for the playwright: the folk-elements may cloud the limited amount of direct political allusion which can be risked. There is always the possibility, therefore, that the audience does not understand the hidden message. This caused Serumaga to further integrate a different kind of folk-element into the plays he wrote after *Majangwa*.

2.2.1.3. *Renga Moi* (1972)

Serumaga's next play was *Renga Moi*. In addition to using legendary material as in *A Play* and *Majangwa*, in *Renga Moi* he also introduced other traditional forms such as music and dance. Obviously, the author tried to reach other Ugandan people in addition to the Baganda with the play, as can be seen in the dialogue which is in four different Ugandan languages, and also by the use of music and dance from several regions.[64] In *Renga Moi*, Serumaga continues his efforts to find an effective way to comment on social and political issues in Uganda without endangering himself. In addition to folk material he applied theatrical techniques developed by Stanislawski, Grotowski and The Living Theatre, thus creating a play filled with emotional images "which aimed at a direct mental association rather than perception by intellectual analysis."[65]

64 Horn, "Individualism and Community," and Mbowa "Ugandan Literature."

65 Serumaga's review of *Renga Moi*, "The Critical Silence," *Uganda Argus*, 3 August 1972, p. 4.

Renga Moi is derived from an Acholi legend from northern Uganda.[66] The chief of the Village of the Seven Hills must choose between defending his village against an attack and completing ritual ceremonies to protect the life of his new-born twins; according to custom, he is not supposed to shed blood during the ceremony. Eventually, he decides to defend his people and risk the life of his twins. During his absence, the village is stricken by privation, so the powerful shaman priest decides to sacrifice the twins to pacify the gods. When Renga Moi, after having won the battle, returns and learns that society, instead of appreciating his sacrifice, has killed his own children, he turns on the priest and kills him.

Renga Moi seems to be Serumaga's clearest statement of his central concern, i.e. the exploration of the decision an individual has to make between personal interests and social commitment.[67] Horn argues that social commitment for Serumaga seems to be an illusory deal. Self-sacrifice is betrayed. Serumaga gives a rather pessimistic outlook on Ugandan society which cannot be saved by the sacrifice of individuals. This attitude stands in clear contrast to Serumaga's own life; he put himself at risk by writing and staging plays that criticised the regime. In 1975, he deemed it advisable to leave the country when he had succeeded in his search for new theatrical forms by producing a rather straight-forward accusation of the Amin-regime with his play *Amanyakiriti*. After three years of exile, he actively joined in the liberation war as commander of a unit.

2.2.1.4. *Amanyakiriti* (1975)

Amanyakiriti is yet another attempt of the author to publicize the mass killings in Uganda. The play was presented at the Commonwealth Writers Conference in 1975. The title of the play is a Kiganda word referring to the bush where dead dogs are thrown and "brought a connotation of death to

---

66 The name 'Renga Moi' has been translated in most articles as 'The Red Warrior' (s. Horn, "Individualism and Community," p. 45). A.C.A. Wright in "Some Notes on Acoli religious Ceremonies," *Uganda Journal*, III, 3, January 1936, explains that "the 'moi' name, which is very highly prized, can be gained by killing any person, male or female, full-grown or a child" (p. 187). The title is adopted at a ceremony, and the new name ends in 'moi,' which is untranslatable. Horn quotes Okot p'Bitek and his discussion of Acoli 'warrior titles' in *The Horn of My Love*, London: Heinemann (AWS 147); Exeter, NH: Heinemann Inc., 1974. P'Bitek explains the title as "Arengo-Moi... one who kills an enemy after hunting him out of the main body" (p. 177).

67 Horn, "Individualism and Community," and Mbowa, "Ugandan Literature."

the audience."[68] As *Renga Moi* before, *Amanyakiriti* communicated through emotional images, only this time there were no words. One character, a dumb man seated next to a coffin, tries to speak. He represents Uganda, unable to speak because of the fear of death. A Kenyan review of the play said that it "appealed to the deepest emotions through mime, dance and song, leaving the audience awestruck and in some cases in tears."[69]

With *Amanyakiriti*, Serumaga again succeeded in making political comments without putting himself into trouble. As Mbowa relates, Amin clearly did not understand the play as a criticism of his rule but actually liked it so much that he invited the group to perform for the OAU-Meeting in 1975. However, since the political statement of the play was straightforward enough, Serumaga decided to go into exile for fear that people who had understood, might speak out.[70]

Serumaga's impact on modern TFD plays is evident and considerable. He tried to disguise political meaning by integrating traditional folkloristic forms in his plays expressing his criticism through the reshaping of legends and customs in order to make it possible for the audience to draw parallels between the play and the political situation of the time. In the earlier plays *A Play* and *Majangwa* where the emphasis was still on narrative traditional forms, the necessity to camouflage the message seems to have been of primary concern. Through the years, when the activities of the Amin-regime became more brutal, the urge to communicate more clearly to the audience led Serumaga to employ other folklore elements, such as music, dance and mime.[71] In his latest play, the message had become so clear that he had to flee into exile.

The way a play is understood and interpreted is determined to a great extent by the spectators' affiliation to a particular culture. This becomes evident when looking at the different interpretations of Serumaga's plays by Rose Mbowa and Andrew Horn. This realization is one of the reasons that has led international organizations nowadays to just sponsor TFD projects and have them carried out by Ugandans. A Theatre for Development play designed by a Ugandan for a Ugandan audience, will communicate more effectively than a play created by outsiders. Members of the same culture

---

68 Mbowa, "Ugandan Literature."

69 quoted in Horn, "Individualism and Community," p. 38.

70 Mbowa, "Ugandan Literature."

71 s. chapter 2.2.2.

know when to allude to common tradition, which gestures to use, which proverbs etc., thus appealing to the audience more efficiently.

Theatre for Development plays that are written and performed today profit from Serumaga's experience. Like him, they convey their message through the use of folkloric elements and thereby refer to the audience's common cultural knowledge. There is, however, an important difference. Today's TFD artists apply that method as a strategy to communicate to the emotions of the spectators and thus convince them. Serumaga, on the other hand, while appealing to audience's emotions, employed folklore in order to disguise his comments on politics - which gives the technique a rather different quality. Today, the strategy of appeal merely helps to create an emotional atmosphere that enhances a sense of belonging and social responsibility. In the course of the play, the spectators come to realise that it is their duty to bring about change for the benefit of the entire community. Like Serumaga, TFD artists have realised that music, dance and mime relate more directly to the audience than narrative forms. They pick up where Serumaga left off in order to convey their didactic messages directly to the audience. Music, dance and mime serve the dual-purpose of entertainment and of conveying a message on an emotional level that does not leave room for misunderstandings.

2.2.2. Nuwa Sentongo

Nevertheless, there are examples for the effective use of narrative folk material. In a play which comments strongly on the Amin regime, Nuwa Sentongo relied on narrative forms when he applied a Ganda myth so relevant to the terror of the time that it could not be misunderstood by Ugandan audiences.

In *The Invisible Bond* (1975), Nuwa Sentongo refers to the Ganda myth of the *Basezi*, the Luganda term for night-dancers. According to Mair, night-dancers are witch-doctors or prowlers who eat human flesh and destroy crops:

> They are human beings who roam by night, clad only in dry banana leaves, or naked, and can be heard hoarsely whispering: 'Wa-wa-wa!' Their main object is to procure human flesh on which to feed; this they do by raising the dead from their graves, by capturing living persons whom they may meet, or even by entering houses and taking people out. In their spare time they amuse

themselves by playing malicious tricks; they pull up crops, cut the seeds, and leave the stalks lying on the ground, knock, or simply kick the door in...[72]

The play begins at night when the *Basezi* are on their way to call the body of Damulira out of his grave. Damulira, however, is rescued from the hands of the night-dancers by Kibaate, and he now clings to Kibaate's back. Kibaate at first has power over Damulira, who relies on being carried since he cannot walk by himself. The relationship changes over time, and Kibaate falls under Damulira's command. In the course of the play, it becomes clear to the audience that Kibaate has killed Damulira by witchcraft because he was the lover of Kibaate's young wife. Kibaate does not know Damulira's true identity until the end of the play, when Damulira forces him to confess his guilt:[73]

Kibaate:	Damulira must die. The Diviner has given me the medicine to kill him.
Corpse:	You told me you love human life.
Kibaate:	Of course I do. I love human life very much but I must safeguard my interests. I love the woman. I can't allow anybody to take her away from me.
Corpse:	Doesn't Damulira love her?
Kibaate:	What does it matter if he loves her? What matters is me. We all love ourselves. We are selfish. I am a victim of human nature, I can't help it. I'm not ashamed of it and I am not going to hide anything. Damulira must die.[74]

While Kibaate and Damulira are in the forest, trying to escape the night-dancers, the *Basezi* trap Kibaate's wife at home. After Kibaate's confession of guilt the night-dancers come in with the corpse of his wife. When she sees the corpse of Damulira she gives him signs of her love. "Stop that," the night-dancers tell them, "Damulira and you are both corpses and we are going to eat you!"[75] The play ends with Kibaate's self-interest being "framed by his society's amoral metaphysical world, peopled by the Night-dancers and the dead whom they devour."[76] The play can be interpreted as a

72 Mair, quoted in Emmanuel Mbogo, "Pre-Capitalist - Pre-Colonial Theater in East Africa: Kenya, Uganda and Tanzania," Diss. Humboldt Universität zu Berlin, 1985. p. 72.

73 Michael Etherton, "Trends in African Theatre," in *African Literature Today. Retrospect & Prospect*, ed. Eldred Durosimi Jones (London, Ibadan, Nairobi: Heinemann, 1979), p. 59.

74 Nuwa Sentongo, *The Invisible Bond*, in Michael Etherton (ed.), *African Plays for Playing*, Vol. 1 (London: Heinemann AWS 165, 1975).

75 *The Invisible Bond*, p. 44.

76 Etherton, "Trends in African Theatre," p. 59.

description of the political situation in Uganda under Amin. The entrapment of Kibaate's innocent wife mirrors the fate of many innocents during Amin's regime of terror.

The belief that witches call out dead bodies is prevalent in many parts of Africa. It is a common myth that they eat the flesh of corpses and take some of the body-parts as ingredients of the most powerful charms. Another reason for resuscitating corpses is to obtain a confidant who can be sent about on evil errands.[77] Night-witches, as night-dancers are also called, are beings who violate every norm and custom considered vital in constituting the identity of society.[78] Among the Baganda and the Lugbara, an ethnic group from western Uganda, there is the belief that witches dance naked. This indicates that night-dancers are to be seen as a projection of evil, since dancing naked is a severe offence against the moral norms of those societies.[79]

In *The Invisible Bond*, Sentongo uses that notion about night-dancers to comment on Idi Amin and on Ugandan society under his regime. To employ a myth related to witchcraft seems particularly appropriate to describe Amin's rule, as he himself was known to be superstitious.[80] Just as Kibaate in the play kills Damulira to get his wife, so had Amin killed the lover of his wife Sarah.

By using the myth of night-dancers in his play, Nuwa Sentongo not only exposes the guilt of Idi Amin the individual, but also that of Ugandan society during the time. In *The Invisible Bond*, the once innocent wives of the night-dancers take to eating bodies, and thereby become involved. Mbowa here sees a direct comment on society during Amin's regime, where "the evil of society is now swallowing up everybody."[81] The self-destructive mechanisms of the man-eat-man society under Amin are exposed in the play when even Kibaate who, through his murder of Damulira has joined

---

77 Alice Werner, *Myths and Legends of the Bantu* (London: Frank Cass, 1968), pp. 247/8.

78 Lucy P. Mair, *Magie im Schwarzen Erdteil* (München: Kindlers Universitätsbibliothek, 1969), pp. 36-42.

79 Mair distinguishes between day- and night-witches. Day-witches are people who are suspected to be witches. They are actual persons living in the community. Very often, they are people who for some reason do not entirely fit in society and are therefore suspected of witchcraft.

80 s. chapter 2.2.1.

81 Mbowa, "Ugandan Literature."

the system, tries to run away from it. Eventually, they are all destroyed by their own network.

When the play was performed in Kampala, it was enthusiastically received by Ugandan audiences. When it was produced in Nigeria, however, to predominantly student audiences, it left them puzzled and bemused, as Michael Etherton reports.[82] He points out that Nuwa Sentongo in the play "shows the way in which the metaphysical way of the Baganda can be used to explore moral behaviour quite independently of Western liberal thought."[83] The play obviously is based on an ethnic background and can only be appreciated in this context. Even though written and performed in English, the major part of the communication process is by images: "The visual references of the forms, like the choreography of the dancers, the masks and the rituals, as well as of the substance, like the religious beliefs and the rites of passage, may be hopelessly inaccessible to people living on the other side of the continent."[84] This again, as already pointed out in the analyses of Serumaga's plays, underlines the necessity for a play to be rooted in the political and social framework of the target audience in order to communicate effectively.

Criticism of Idi Amin's regime was however not the only subject of Ugandan theatre before 1986. In the next two chapters, plays criticising the two Obote regimes will be discussed, all of which again use folklore to address the issues of the time.

2.2.3. Byron Kawadwa

Byron Kawadwa, one of the most famous playwrights of the 1970s in Uganda, was director of the National Theatre in Kampala until his murder by Amin's security police in 1977. Kawadwa had been involved in theatrical activities since secondary school. It was in school where he encountered western style theatre through Shakespeare performances on Parents' Day. His early exposure to drama and theatre eventually inspired him to organise the School Drama Festival.[85] In 1964 he founded the Kampala City Players, a non-professional group, whose members worked as civil servants or

82 Etherton, "Trends in African Theatre," p. 58.

83 ibid., p. 58.

84 ibid., p. 59.

85 Breitinger, "Popular Urban Theatre," p. 270.

traders during the day and only performed in the evenings. Kawadwa, together with his former teacher, Wycliff Kyingi, and the musician Wassanyi Serukenya, became famous for creating musical plays, which were performed in Luganda and used traditional settings.[86] He worked for Radio Uganda, when, during the Emergency after Obote's republican confrontation with the hereditary Kabaka of Buganda, he was arrested and detained without trial. After his release, he could not reclaim his post with Radio Uganda, and began to concentrate on theatre. His most outstanding plays are *Makula ga Kulabako* and *Oluyimba lwa Wankoko* (*The Song of Wankoko*), where he "combined acute social observation, a deep affection for the culture of his native Buganda, a keen sense of stage spectacle, and Serukenya's rich musical scores for traditional Kiganda instruments, to produce neatly patterned romantic comedies."[87]

In 1976, *The Song Of Wankoko* represented Uganda at the 'Festival of Black and African Arts and Culture' (FESTAC) in Lagos/Nigeria. It was performed under the direction of playwright Elvania Zirimu for an international audience. Before leaving for Lagos, Kawadwa received permission to stage again his play *Saint Lwanga*. The play, which was first produced in 1969 for the visit of Pope Paul VI to Uganda, tells the story of the Ugandan Martyrs, a group of twenty-two Baganda Catholics. They were burned to death in June 1885 by Kabaka Mwanga, at the counsel of his Arab adviser Salim bin Juma.[88]

During Kawadwa's absence, resistance against the Amin regime grew at home. Ugandan exile groups carried out sabotage missions against Amin, and the Church also began to raise its voice in protest. In January 1977 Amin and his advisers decided to crush the mounting opposition. An army of killer squads moved through the country and massacred civilians. All areas suffered, but the main focus of the attack was on Acholi and Langi. This was the situation which led to the murder of Archbishop Luwum, an Acholi, in February 1977, while Kawadwa was still in Lagos. One Saturday morning, 5 February 1977, Amin's soldiers came to the Archbishop's house and searched it. Following that incident, bishops, assistant bishops, and the Archbishop himself wrote an open letter of protest. Seven days later, on 17 February 1977, Radio Uganda announced the death of Archbishop Luwum,

86 Horn, "Individualism and Community."

87 Andrew Horn, "Uganda's Theatre - the Exiled and the Dead," *Index on Censmrship*, 8/5 (1979), pp. 12-15.

88 ibid.

immediately causing world-wide protests against religious persecution in Uganda.[89] When Kawadwa, after his return, resumed rehearsals of *Saint Lwanga*, a play about the slaughter of Christians, this must have appeared like a direct accusation to the Muslim regime of Idi Amin.

In early March 1977, Kawadwa was dragged by men of Amin's State Research Bureau from rehearsals at the National Theatre. Five days later, his body, along with those of five other members of the *Saint Lwanga* cast, was found in a forest near Kampala. The real reasons for his death can only be speculated upon; it might have been ordered as a consequence of his theatre work or possibly because he had been abroad and was consequently suspected of subversive activities and cooperation with anti-Amin groups. Ironically, his most outstanding play was not *Saint Lwanga*, but *The Song of Wankoko* which was performed at FESTAC in 1976.

2.2.3.1. *The Song Of Wankoko*

The play is about Wankoko who, together with his companion Nkwale, comes to the King's Palace where he attempts to oust the King and become the leader of the maladministrated Kingdom himself. Soon after his arrival at the palace, he tries to make the palace-workers realise the oppression they are suffering under the present system. Meanwhile he befriends Prince Suuna, who is in love with Princess Barungi, but is too shy to declare his love to her. Wankoko is supposed to court her in the Prince's name, but rather than doing that, he declares his own love for her. Eventually, he falsely accuses the Prince of treachery and the King banishes Suuna. Wankoko now hopes to marry the Princess, thus raising himself to the ranks of the aristocracy. Princess Barungi follows Suuna, whom she still loves, into exile in the forest. There, the Prince finally gives proof of his braveness and courage by fearlessly fighting wild animals. Princess Barungi succeeds in convincing the King of Suuna's innocence, and the play ends with Barungi's and Suuna's marriage.

With *The Song Of Wankoko*, Kawadwa created a play which even today attracts large audiences. The combined use of folklore elements of song and dance, together with Serukenya's music seem to appeal immediately not only to Baganda, but to international audiences as well - albeit on different intellectual, emotional and cultural levels. For a Ugandan audience, the

89 Wooding and Barnett, *Uganda Holocaust*, p. 20.

play has a deeper meaning; through it's use of music, dance, and a story about a Baganda King, the play makes a socio-political comment on Obote's coming to power and the abolition of the Kingdoms. There are clear parallels between Wankoko's actions in the play and Obote's actions in reality.

In Kawadwa's play, Wankoko introduces himself with a song to the palace workers who take it up as chorus, thereby giving it the form of traditional Bantu folk songs:

> My name is indeed Wankoko
> I came in hearing that you had problems
> Your problems are my problems
> What pleases you pleases me as well.
> Now let me tell you why they call me Wankoko
> I spend all my time in moving up and down
> the country searching for trouble-spots
> Trying to help the oppressed and helpless
> And by the time I leave such places
> It is happiness all around.[90]

In that first song, the audience is given hints about the true character of Wankoko, who "does not respect the dignity of labour."[91] His name, which is the Luganda word for cock, implies the loud animal that only scratches towards itself - and Wankoko turns out to be selfish. He does not hesitate to court Princess Barungi himself in order to rise socially and gain influence, although with that action he betrays both Prince Suuna and the palace workers who have elected him as their leader.

In his song, Wankoko implies that there is oppression in the palace, and in the next few scenes, he tries to make the palace workers aware of that oppression. Before he came, they had been content with their subordination under the King and accepted the social system. Their love for the King is reinforced in their song:

> We are the King's men
> Ready to do anything at his bidding...
> We are the King's maids
> Ready to fulfill all his wishes...
> Together through all hardships and battles
> We are not weaklings

90 Byron Kawadwa and Wessanyi Serukenya, *The Song of Wankoko* (Kampala: Ministry of Culture and Community Development, 1977), p. 1-2.

91 Mercy Mirembe, "The Influence of Ugandan Folklore on Ugandan Theatre," MA-thesis, Makerere University, Kampala/Uganda, 1990, p. 221

Bullied by whoever comes along...
We all give support to our King
Like drunkards drenched in their drink
We are a people steeped in love for our
King...
the King, our King deserves all our gratitude
The gratitude we bestow upon a rainstorm
Which on pausing allows travellers to get
to their destinations...
We are the King's men.
We are the King's maids.
Ready to die for our King.[92]

In another song, however, Wankoko, now also a palace worker, teaches them that all men are created equal:

An insect is created like an insect
An animal is created like an animal
A bird is created like a bird
And man is created like man
Thus an insect is treated like an insect
And an animal is treated like an animal
A bird is treated like a bird
And man is treated like man.[93]

Eventually, all the workers join him as chorus. A Ugandan audience, aware of the parallel between Wankoko and Obote, clearly sees the connection between the song, "Man is Man," and Obote's Common Man's Charter.[94] A similar parallel is drawn later in the play, depicting Obote's conflict with the King: Wankoko disregards the custom that prohibits people from squatting in the palace. This can be interpreted as a social protest against administrative oppression, like Obote's 1967 disregard for the federal structure of Uganda when he introduced the republican constitution and abolished the rule of traditional leaders.[95]

In the next scene, Nkwale enters with a little drum campaigning openly for Wankoko to become the leader of the palace guards. After the palace guards have been thus prepared for the elections, Wankoko comes in. In the 1990 production of the play at the National Theatre in Kampala (by Nyonza Singers) Wankoko enters the stage giving the popular UPC hand wave, thus

92 *The Song of Wankoko*, p. 3-4.

93 *The Song of Wankoko*, p. 14.

94 s. Mirembe, "The Influence of Ugandan Folklore."

95 ibid., p. 229.

showing the connection between himself and Obote.[96] In a speech he claims that he has solutions to the workers' problems. Nonetheless, at first only a few of the palace guards raise their hands to vote for him; he nevertheless prevails, reminding the audience of the way Obote supplanted the 1962 Constitution and put his republican Constitution in place:[97]

> Alright, put your hands up everybody. (all the workers raise their hands). Good! that's it. Thank you very much for giving me your support.[98]

The palace workers, in their willingness to follow Wankoko, constitute the ruled Ugandans under Obote. By showing in a satirical manner how Wankoko manipulates their vote, and how easily they are manipulated, the playwrights criticise the ready acceptance of Obote's 1966 Republican Constitution by the Ugandan population. Wankoko, like Obote, had manipulated and indoctrinated the population by seemingly liberating society from oppression. As it turned out, however, he merely advanced his own political ambitions.

Prince Suuna clearly stands for Kabaka Muteesa who was ousted by Obote. Especially towards the end of the play, when Prince Suuna is in 'exile' in the forest, wearing Muteesa's hunting attire, Ugandans recognise their former King who died in exile.

One reason for the continuing popularity of the play is its rich use of folklore elements. The costumes are reminiscent of the time when Buganda was still a kingdom, and even today, this has an emotional impact on the spectators - many of whom still lament the loss of the monarchy. The figure of Wankoko itself is folkloristic. He represents the trickster character common in African folktales, who is known not only in the Ugandan folk-tradition, but throughout the continent.[99]

The songs and dances integrated in the play are reminiscent of traditional folksongs, and like them, regulate the spectators' anxieties, curiosities and tension.[100] Kawadwa and Serukenya changed the traditional pattern, however, and filled it with new meaning. The songs' structure resembles those of Ganda folk-songs, but they go a step further in that they do not always follow the basic repetitious pattern. Quite often, the rhythm is

[96] ibid.

[97] s. chapter 2.2.1.

[98] *The Song of Wankoko*, p. 14.

[99] Mirembe, "The Influence of Ugandan Folklore," p. 250.

[100] ibid.

changed to better communicate Wankoko's propaganda. Most of the songs, for example, do not have the simplistic form typical for folk-songs. They extend beyond the usual three to six lines of a traditional folk music stanza before a refrain or stanza is repeated.[101] The songs with their familiar structure now serve to communicate Wankoko's propaganda to the palace workers. They also convey to the audience the connection between Wankoko and Obote, and with it, the criticism of Obote's actions.

Like Serumaga and Sentongo, Byron Kawadwa also employs elements from Ganda folklore to convey his criticism on political events. There is an important difference, however. Whereas for Serumaga and Sentongo, it was a potentially life-saving device to hide their criticism, for Kawadwa in *The Song of Wankoko* it was a purely artistic technique. Kawadwa wrote the play as criticism on the Obote I regime, when Amin, having ousted Obote, was already president. There was no immediate danger in criticising Obote's government. The author therefore could, quite unlike Serumaga and Sentongo, afford to write a play that is much more accessible to the audience than *A Play* or *The Invisible Bond*. The structure is simpler, and the reason for using folk-material is clearly not to disguise the message, but to bring it across more effectively. This is also the motive of present-day TFD artists when they apply folklore. In most plays, we find Kawadwa's/Serukenya's idea of taking up folk songs or rather their tunes, because they are familiar to the audience. As in the *Song of Wankoko*, the words are changed to convey a certain message. Kawadwa's impact on TFD therefore, is more direct than that of Serumaga and Sentongo since he applied the same techniques for the purpose of communicating more effectively.

2.2.4. Fagil Mandy

Fagil Mandy, who in his play *Endless Night* deals critically with Obote's handling of the election campaign in 1980, could not risk to communicate as directly as Kawadwa.[102] Just as Serumaga and Sentongo, he camouflaged his political criticism for his own safety. He developed new ways of conveying information to the audience, mainly absurdist techniques, but he

---

[101] ibid., p. 251.

[102] *Endless Night*, unpublished, was Mandy's script for 3rd year BA and BA (Educ) in his Drama Majors' examination in Playwriting and Production at MDD/Makerere University.

also retained dramatic forms of the older playwrights, such as folklore elements. This indicates that to communicate effectively to a Ugandan audience references to folklore are seen to be necessary.

The play depicts the story of the blind beggar Kafa. Every day, he sits in the streets in his wheel-barrow hoping to get some money from passers-by who would feel pity for him. All he gets, however, is abuse. He and his crippled wife place all their hopes in their only child, a son. On the other side of the stage, the rich are shown; here are Ronny and his wife Stella who carries a bundle that seems to be a baby. Eventually, however, it is revealed that Ronny, after an accident, has become impotent. The wife nurses a doll to maintain the illusion that she has a child. At the end of the play, when the doll is crushed, she has to accept the fact that she is without a baby. The son of the beggars goes with Stella and Ronny, leaving his parents alone and without hope.

The play examines human situations from childhood through youth to old age and death;[103] it is also a criticism of the 1980 general election in Uganda. In *Endless Night*, Mandy develops Serumaga's complicated structures even further. He uses absurdist techniques to convey his criticism on the current political events. The action takes place on five rostri arranged in a circle symbolising various human states: Kafa's home is at rostrum no. 3, his begging place at rostrum no. 2; on rostrum no. 1, Kafa's memories are enacted; rostrum no. 4 is Ronnie's home, and on rostrum no. 5 his and Stella's marriage is enacted.

The beggar in the play implies the view of Obote's opponents that the "rigged ballots after heavy 'begging' during campaigns"[104] helped Obote in assuming the presidency of Uganda for a second time.[105] Significantly, the action takes place on rostri, usually a place where political speeches are held. Kafa, the blind beggar, is seated in a black wheel-barrow with the inscription 'Endless Night.' The inscription and the play's title allude to the author's message, i.e. the blind and crippled beggar, who lives in eternal darkness, represents the situation Uganda found itself in after the elections. People had hoped for free elections, and after 1980 those hopes were

---

103 for a more detailed discussion, s. Mirembe, "The Influence of Ugandan Folklore," pp. 369-406.

104 ibid., p. 372.

105 Fagil Mandy was a member of the Uganda Peoples Movement (UPM), led by Yoweri Museveni. UPM was one of the parties that were defeated in the elections. Mandy today holds a high position in the NRM-Secretariate.

repeatedly crushed. Uganda seemed to drag along as if in an endless night.[106] This is exemplified in a scene when a well-dressed lady passes Kafa in the street without bothering to give him anything. Kafa comments on her behaviour:

> Seeming to be hurrying somewhere. To get something for herself maybe. Well! And my day so long seems to be hurrying to an unsuccessful end.[107]

Mirembe here draws a convincing parallel to the socio-political background of the play. That the lady hurries somewhere to 'get' something for herself, while the beggar is uncertain of what the day will provide for him, shows that "Kafa typifies the feeling of the 'crippled' political contestors towards those who knew what they were getting out of the game."[108] In another scene, the empty promises of the politicians during the campaign are exposed even more openly, when "pop music blares up, and a group of young men and women, old men and old women, emerges from stage left dancing with abandon... in various ways of promiscuity bordering on grotesqueness."[109] One of the dancers, acting as politician, climbs onto rostrum no. 2 and promises his listeners free education, free health services, homes for the aged, and liberation of the poor, if they vote him into power.[110] As they go out, each of the dancers spits at Kafa, "typifying the loss of morals and human values during the political campaigns (rallies)."[111] The scene is a comment on Obote's promises during the campaigns which were forgotten as soon as he had assumed power.

Among all the plays discussed so far, *Endless Night* is the play that makes the least use of folklore although folk-elements are found in the plotting of man's life cycle and in the songs in local languages. As with the other playwrights, Fagil Mandy seems to be convinced that folklore is the appropriate medium to bring across his message to the spectators. It is familiar to most members of the audience and also has an emotional impact. The appeal to tradition creates a sense of togetherness thereby making the audience more favourably disposed to accept the play's viewpoint.

---

106 Mbowa, "Ugandan Literature."

107 *Endless Night*, p. 1.

108 Mirembe, "The Influence of Ugandan Folklore," p. 375.

109 *Endless Night*, p. 5.

110 Mirembe, "The Influence of Ugandan Folklore," p. 380.

111 ibid., p. 381.

The aforementioned plays represent attempts at political comment of artists during two decades of oppressive regimes in Uganda. It must be stressed that these attempts were few in number and eventually had to be stopped, especially after Kawadwa was killed and Serumaga had gone into exile. Nonetheless, their influence on present-day TFD prevails. In didactic plays about health education we still find communicative strategies developed by the literary dramatists. While handling folklore in different ways, all the playwrights share a dynamic approach to tradition: the authors took old familiar forms and filled them with new meaning. This dynamic use of folklore and tradition probably constitutes the most important contribution of the political dramatists to present-day Theatre for Development. As will be seen in the discussion of the case studies, there are various ways in which the fight against AIDS is tackled through theatre. Artists producing a play with the primary aim of communicating their message about how to prevent the infection with AIDS adopt the dynamic approach of the literary artists by filling familiar folklore forms with new meaning; they try to both educate and entertain their audiences. There are other artists, however, who present the topic AIDS on stage by employing popular art forms in a static way, merely repeating old forms. An example would be the presentation of traditional dances in an urban centre like Kampala by JK Ebonita.[112] They practice what Desai calls de-popularisation, since "they display normative rearticulations without effecting corresponding changes in formalistic terms."[113] When dealing with a topic like AIDS using those art forms, their concern is not really AIDS education. They are rather commercially and psychologically motivated by entertaining the urban elite and reassuring "the developing nation that it has not ignored its national culture."[114]

The regimes of Obote and Amin between 1966 and 1985 eventually made it increasingly difficult for politically and socially committed theatre to exist. Those theatre activities that still flourished were the presentation of drawing-room comedy and light entertainment.[115] Some of the committed theatrical groups continued to exist in name, but nobody tried to explore new forms to convey meaning. This fact also has to do with the audiences.

---

112 for a detailed discussion of Ebonita's productions. s. chapter 4.3.

113 Desai, "Theater as Praxis," p. 68.

114 ibid., p. 68.

115 for further information about urban popular plays, s. Breitinger, "Popular Urban Theatre," pp. 270-290.

During the years of oppression an increasing number of intellectuals left the country and went into exile. Other East African intellectuals, who had contributed to the flourishing of Makerere University, also turned their backs on Uganda.[116] There was no intellectual audience left that would have appreciated technically complex plays like *Majangwa* or *Endless Night*. The audience that remained was not looking for plays that would remind them of the oppression they were suffering. They wanted escapism, not social commentary. Theatre remained non-committal until the political climate in Uganda changed.

2.3. Theatre after 1986

In 1986, the National Resistance Army under Yoweri Museveni won the liberation war and built a Government committed to the observation of human rights and freedom of speech. Suddenly, in and around Kampala, numerous theatrical groups emerged. With the change in the political situation, however, the forms of theatre could no longer remain the same as in the sixties and seventies. Since the Indians were expelled in 1972 by Amin, and the expatriate population left the country, it became harder to draw demarcation lines between cultural interests along ethnic lines. As Breitinger demonstrates, theatrical activities before the civil war were organized according to ethnic divisions: there were African, Asian, and expatriate theatre groups, each catering for their own specific audiences.[117] Social stratification in post-war Ugandan society changed, and with it the cultural activities. The comedies that existed throughout the civil war, are still performed and are still popular. But there are now numerous TFD-activities, for the NRM Government makes an effort to monitor the redefinition and rebirth of social and cultural needs and aspirations. This also means that an open political climate promotes the flourishing of different forms of theatre. The President has called on Ugandans to help in the reconstruction of the country. Theatre plays a part here as a powerful instrument for educating the people and affecting change in support of the development of the country. The importance of Theatre for Development in Uganda becomes evident when one bears in mind that forty-eight percent of the population is illiterate, and most people do not have access to television. In such a situation, a combination of public lectures and theatre/video in

[116] ibid.

[117] ibid., p. 273.

rural and urban areas serves the need for both entertainment and information. Although it is only for the last five years that theatre has been used extensively as an instrument of information, there are reports of single projects going back as far as the 1940s. In the following, a brief outline of the history of TFD in Uganda will be given in order to situate present day CT in its historical context.

2.3.1. Theatre for Development in Uganda

Margaret Macpherson reports during the late forties and early fifties, colonial administrators organized educative theatre plays.[118] The concepts and scripts of the plays were designed by the colonial administration in Kampala, and from there they were taken to target groups in rural areas. As Breitinger remarks, this is a very early example of TFD, with "a clear cut top-down strategy of communication."[119] The plays of the 'Mobile Theatre' were mostly related to problems of health, theft and general social behaviour.

Geoffrey Wadulo points out that in addition to the 'Mobile Theatre' there were also Women Development Programmes, designed to enhance women's social and economic development. These programmes were carried out at social centres, and women were instructed about nutritional matters for children and family planning. At the same time, a number of moral issues was discussed.[120]

Another attempt at TFD, although in a broader sense, was the Makerere Travelling Theatre of the 1960s. As the name implies, a group of lecturers and students from the university intended to take theatre to the people. The plays they performed, however, had no development messages; usually the group chose European classics, African plays, and new productions created by their own members.[121] The languages in which they performed were English, Swahili, Luganda, and Runyoro/Rutoro. Breitinger correctly points out that the plays were educative nevertheless

---

[118] Margaret Macpherson, "Plays and People."

[119] ibid., p. 1.

[120] s.a. Geoffrey Wadulo, "'Theatre for Development' in Uganda," unpublished research report, 1990, p. 1.

[121] David Cook, "Theatre Goes to the People!" *Transition*, Vol. 5, no. 25, 1966.

insofar as theatre and cultural activities in general have a morally uplifting or ethically formative effect on the spectators.[122]

TFD activities, just as political theatre, came to an end during the regimes of Milton Obote (1966-1971; 1980-1985) and Idi Amin (1971-1979). In two decades of turmoil, the social and economic infrastructures in the country were destroyed. People were no longer interested in developing the country; they were preoccupied with survival.[123]

Following the end of the Civil War in 1986, in the urban center of Kampala, "social division and the corresponding cultural aspirations seems to have developed in bifocal direction."[124] On the one hand, there is the newly established business community of educated businessmen, merchants, consultants, professionals. Those groups have a commercial ethos. On the other hand, there are slum-dwellers, small traders, hawkers, sellers, the un- and underemployed, among them refugees from the war areas in Eastern- and Southern Buganda, as well as North- and North-Eastern Uganda. They are more interested in survival than commercial success. I think Breitinger is right when he assumes that theatrical and cultural activities are now geared along lines of socio-economical rather than ethnic division. The various theatrical groups still cater for their specific audiences, just as had been done previously, but the specifics have changed; especially in the field of Theatre for Development, this means that "the role of the intellectuals as founders, managers, motors of cultural and theatrical groups with socio-cultural-political intentions, has now been taken over by often ideologically motivated, politically committed, humanitarean oriented groups and individuals from government ministries (in particular Health and Education) or from the various non-governmental organizations (NGO) like UNICEF, World Health Organization, Red Cross, Mothers Union etc..."[125]

Since 1986, health education, i.e. information about diarrhoeal diseases, immunization, and more recently AIDS prevention, as well as the prevention of other sexually transmitted diseases, has become of primary concern. Consequently, most TFD plays today, sponsored by either GOs, or NGOs focus on those topics. Until the last two to three years, the emphasis in Theatre for Development was not so much on nationwide information

---

[122] Breitinger, "Popular Urban Theatre," p. 271.

[123] Wadulo, "'Theatre for Development' in Uganda."

[124] Breitinger, "Popular Urban Theatre."

[125] ibid., p. 272.

campaigns. Instead, projects concentrated on one area and through theatre tried to implement concrete development goals. In the following sub-chapters, some of those projects will be described. The focus of the description will be on the organizational and methodological side of the projects rather than on the dramatic techniques applied in the plays. This is done, because TFD by its very nature involves more than just the theatrical event of the performance.[126] The discussion of organization and implementation of the projects will also shed some light on the significance of the organizational framework as it has developed in CT today.

2.3.1.1. Jonathan Muganga's Nattyole Project (1986)

Muganga is an alumni of the Department of Music, Dance and Drama (MDD) at Makerere University and now works with the Ministry of Health. In 1986, Vicencia Sserwadda, an Agricultural Officer/Nutritionist, planned to introduce a Primary Health Care project in Nattyole. The project was to be sponsored by a non-governmental organization (NGO), the Catholic Secretariate, a subsidiary of the Catholic Church. Nattyole is a village in Luweero district, popularly known as 'Luweero Triangle.' As in most villages in the area, a large percentage of Nattyole's population was killed by Obote's army in attacks on presumed guerilla fighters. After 1986, villagers who had fled the district began to return; many suffered from diseases like Kwashiorkor, hookworm aneamia, diahhroea, dysentery, scabies and malaria, which were exacerbated by ignorance and bad living conditions.

Morale in the village was so low, however, that few people attended Ms. Sserwadda's sessions and lectures. She began looking for somebody more experienced in social mobilization to give the project a proper start. Jonathan Muganga had already had experience with Primary Health Care; he decided to help initiate the project and use it as a research activity for MDD and the Health Education Division of the Ministry of Health.[127]

The goal of the project was to implement Primary Health Care as a practical and economical way of improving the standard of health in the community. The plan was to have Nattyole as centre for the project from where, at a later stage, the message was supposed to spread to neighbouring

---

[126] for a definition of TFD, s. Introduction.

[127] Jonathan Muganga, "Theatre for Development in Uganda. The Nattyole Experience," (Ministry of Health [Uganda] Health Education Division) unpublished research report, 1990, p. 1.

villages. Sserwadda and Muganga wanted to act as catalysts assisting the people in taking on "an active share, role and responsibility in shaping their own lives and development. This was through 'Theatre for Development,' which turned out to be the Project eye-opener."[128]

The Project was carried out in cooperation with the Catholic Church, on whose premises the meetings took place. For the first meeting, six women from the village turned up. Muganga considered this a promising start. To increase their self-confidence, they formed a club. Together, the club members and the initiators formulated the objectives of their project:

- Identification of health and other social problems
- Prioritization of the problems
- Causes
- Possible remedies to the problems identified
- Community mobilization activities

During their first sessions, five major problems in the village were identified. They were malnutrition among children under five years, death of children from the six vaccine diseases, diarrhoeal diseases, alcoholism among men, and poverty. The club members usually met on Saturdays, and during those meetings, they composed plays with simple stories, poems, and songs. They wanted to create an awareness among their fellow-villagers for problems affecting the whole community.[129]

Muganga relates that their first play dealt with the topic 'Proper Nutrition - a key to development.' The emphasis lay on addressing parents who believe that symptoms of malnutrition are caused by witchcraft. In the production, an attempt was made to clear misconceptions about malnutrition and give information about a balanced diet for children. The issue of men selling family food to buy alcohol was also discussed. Mothers were asked to join the club in order to get more information. At the end of the play, the women sang a song, 'Endiisa' (Feeding) to emphasize their message.[130]

After the performance of the first production, more plays, poems, songs were created. They discussed other problems, such as the treatment of diarrhoeal diseases. As Muganga stresses, emphasis was laid on "simple, familiar, acceptable words in the community, and also on logical, clear,

---

[128] ibid., p. 4.

[129] ibid., p. 7.

[130] ibid., p. 7.

precise and conclusive messages avoiding unnecessary information but maintaining entertainment and interest."[131]

The plays were advertised through places of worship, Resistance Council Meetings,[132] and schools. This was done so effectively that many people came to attend the performances, and eventually the club grew larger and could create more plays. The community began to appreciate the work of the club and donated money so that costumes could be bought. Fame spread and there were invitations by Bishops of the Catholic Church to perform in Hoima and Kampala. By that time, the club had enough members to establish further groups who would go to neighbouring villages and spread the message there.[133] At home, concerts and dinners for the group members were held to further discussions and the exchange of knowledge.

The project evolved so well that it even had a measurable economic impact. The club members established a demonstration garden on land of the Catholic Parish Church in order to show how to plant crops necessary for a balanced diet. This caused still more people to develop an interest in the club activities. Eventually, the club members grew similar crops at home, and the surplus was sold. The same was done with handicraft, and they even started animal husbandry, which also brought them some money and in turn encouraged other members of the community to join the project. A co-operative society was established, and what had started as a Primary Health Care Campaign, developed into an agricultural project for the benefit of the whole community. All the while, however, the health education activities continued.[134]

Muganga's project is discussed in detail here, because it appears to me that, unlike many of the nationwide campaigns we see today, it had an approach to the solution of the problems of communities that almost automatically ensured its success. Contrary to the big campaigns it focussed on one small area, and from there it spread to other places in the district.

---

131 ibid., p. 8.

132 Since the NRM under Yoweri Museveni came to power in 1986, the political organization of the country is divided up into the so-called Resistance Councils. The councils are on different levels, such as RC I at the district and village level, up to RC V. The structure is supposed to ensure maximum and direct participation of the Ugandan population in political decisions.

133 By the end of the fifth month the number of interested members had grown to over 30. s.a. Muganga, "The Nattyole Experience," p. 9.

134 ibid., p. 10.

The focus on one locality made it possible to address issues in a way that was oriented towards the target-group's needs and habits. The plays did not have to remain unspecific in the presentation of the problems and thus gained deeper relevance for the people in the area. The whole community was actively involved and therefore interested in the project's success. Before Muganga started the project, he talked to the priest of the local Catholic Church, elders, women leaders, a teacher and RC leaders, thus involving the influential people of the area through whom he could advertise his project effectively. It is important to reiterate that Muganga and Ms. Sserwadda only served as catalysts. In the plays, villagers themselves identified their problems, made a problem analysis, and created plays and songs in which they suggested solutions. Club members became involved in health education work to change people's attitudes and inform them about child immunization, protected drinking water, safe sexual behaviour to prevent AIDS, hygiene, oral rehydration therapy, child education etc.[135] Once they joined the project, they recognised their role in society by reshaping and improving their own living conditions. Through their work on the first play, they eventually gained the awareness that they were indeed able to influence their own community and to solve many of its problems without much outside assistance.

In the Nattyole project, TFD turned out to be an effective impetus to encourage community participation in solving problems effecting the community. By having problem identification, problem analysis, the creation and performance of the plays, as well as the discussion about the solutions to the problems come from the villagers themselves, they were able to use "community channels of communication and respected folk artists and communicators in their own community."[136] The Nattyole project is proof that TFD is able to create a consciousness that encourages communities to initiate their own projects. Through theatre, the people of Nattyole have come to the realization that they are the ones to influence their own life.

Although the focus in recent TFD obviously is on nationwide campaigns, there are still projects like Muganga's centred in small communities.

---

135 ibid, p. 10.

136 Muganga, "The Nattyole Experience," p. 11.

2.3.1.2. Geoffrey Wadulo's Project

More recently, a TFD-project similar to Muganga's was carried out by Geoffrey Wadulo, a drama major in Makerere. In 1990, the *Committee for International Self-Reliance* (CIS), an NGO, organised a conference on the 'Promotion of Health in Rural Communities in Uganda,' which was supposed to include a play. Since the conference affected the rural people, Wadulo suggested that the play should also be performed by them.[137] The people from CIS agreed and financed his project. The conference was to take place at Mukono, and as a target group Ntawo was identified, a village about five kilometers away. Wadulo met with those people from Ntawo village who were interested, mostly women and children, and discussed their problems. Again, it appeared that problems related to health seemed most urgent: immunisation, high incidence of diarrhoeal diseases, poor sanitation and unclean drinking water. The people who had turned up for the discussion created a play that was performed at the conference on May 15th 1990. As with Muganga's project in Nattyole, the problem identification and analysis in Ntawo came from the target-group. They created their own play, with Wadulo assisting where necessary.

The first part of the play presents the Mujama family as an example of mistaken behaviour. The name Mujama which is the Luganda word for 'dirty,' implies that their house is dirty, they do not boil their drinking water, the children do not bathe, they are not immunised, their diet is bad. Only one of the many children, a boy, goes to school. Due to his unsettled home, however, he has no place to study. Mr. Mujama neglects his family and spends the little money they have on drink. One day the school-boy collapses with high fever. Mrs. Mujama takes him to hospital where the doctor diagnozes tetanus. The illness could have been avoided had the boy been immunized. Due to negligence and bad treatment by the hospital staff he dies on the way home. Two days later, another child of the family dies from diarrhoea, caused by the dirty living conditions at home. Neighbours and Health Educators come to sympathise and they educate the Mujamas about the dangers of not immunising the children, drinking unboiled water and not using a pit-latrine. The first part of the play ends with the Mujamas singing a song of repentance. The second part shows them in a completely different home: it is clean, and general hygiene is taken seriously.[138]

---

[137] Wadulo, "'Theatre for Development' in Uganda," p. 4.

[138] ibid., p. 8-9.

As a result of the play, it was decided during the conference to build a clinic in Ntawo village, and to start the protection of three water supplies. As in Muganga's project, in Ntawo theatre served as an instrument to show the villagers how to improve their own living conditions. Through theatre, an awareness of their ability to achieve change was created, once they take the initiative and become active.

Wadulo today works as cultural coordinator for the CIS and tries, through TFD, to change the attitude of the people towards development.[139] His target areas now are five of the slum-areas in Kampala (Kibuli, Namuwongo, Kisugi, Makerere Kivulu and Bwaise). The major problem people face in these areas is, as in many other parts of Uganda, a lack of proper sanitation and the associated problems that come with it. In the slums, Wadulo performs plays together with the inhabitants, similar to the one in Ntawo village. The aim is to educate people about the importance of adhering to principles of general hygiene, such as the building of pit-latrines and proper waste-disposal. Follow-up actions, like the building of new pit-latrines, are financed by CIS.

It appears that one of the reasons for the success of Wadulo's and Muganga's projects is that they lead to concrete improvements. People see a play depicting a certain problem, discuss solutions, and then turn the results into reality. Besides the solution to the immediate problem depicted in the play, they also acquire the knowledge to transfer that line of action to other problems in the community. The plays themselves are composed according to that principle: the wrong kind of behaviour is usually shown in the first scene; followed by the negative consequences resulting from that behaviour. The solution is presented in the third scene. Plays such as those carried out by Muganga and Wadulo, which discuss primary health and sanitation problems and are focussed on a comparatively small area have the same pattern as concrete project-oriented plays with the target-group articulating a problem and participating in finding a solution for it. Projects developing health care, however, go a step further than purely project-oriented plays. They do not end with the building of a pit latrine. People are educated about hygiene, and they are now able to transfer their newly acquired knowledge to other health-/hygiene related problems. Their awareness about their ability to act has grown as a direct result of the play. Direct effects of the plays are ensured because the information given in the play is

---

[139] ibid., p. 9.

reinforced by concrete action from outside enabling the people to put their newly acquired knowledge to immediate use. This is contrary to theatre for raising consciousness, such as TFD about AIDS, which is solely concerned with creating awareness and does not have any immediate impact.

2.3.1.3. Rural TFD - The "Crude Theatre" of Kibingo-Village, Bugahya Subcounty, Hoima District

The form of TFD which is the subject of this study, i.e. Campaign Theatre, takes place mainly in the urban centres in the south. The reason for this is that with TFD in Uganda today, there is a special emphasis on topics related to health, especially the prevention of sexually transmitted diseases (STDs) and AIDS. Health education, however, differs from the project oriented plays usually performed in rural areas, which rely on resources available within the community itself: participatory research to identify the problems and organising the human, financial and material resources of the community can be achieved through development theatre activities with relatively little help from outside.[140] Health issues, however, require help from outside, especially when more than just information is needed. Problem analysis and health education can only be carried out responsibly by medically trained personel, expertise not normally available in the villages: "the transmission of health information requires 'translators,' mediators, and especially facilitators who can dispose of organizational, financial, and managerial resources effectively to launch health information campaigns, liaising between medical experts and the actors and performers, and between both of those and the target audience."[141] Due to the emphasis on health issues, TFD in Uganda today necessarily takes place mainly in the urban centres in the south with their accumulation of medical personel and hospitals. Besides, the population density in those areas also causes a higher incidence of health risks and, consequently, a higher demand for health education.

There is, however, an example of a rural Theatre for Development group in the north-west of Uganda which does not practice the project-oriented kind of TFD usually found in rural areas. In the following, I will describe the group's activities in relative detail, because they exemplify the extent to which TFD involves areas that go beyond the purely theatrical

---

140 Breitinger, "Popular Urban Theatre," p. 282.

141 ibid., p. 283.

event. Jessica Kaahwa reports on a group consisting mainly of young people in her home district of Hoima.[142] As early as 1981, the young people in the area started forming a Youth Club for the purpose of mass mobilization through drama. One of their first actions was to disseminate information about the 1980/81 elections. Originally, they were neutral, but by 1983, they started to divide into political groups, depending on the leaders' affiliation to a political party, the non-conformist groups eventually getting banned or arrested. After 1985, with the fall of the Obote-Government, the politicised youth wings also disappeared. Even before 1985, they had stopped referring to the political situation in their plays. The atmosphere towards the end of the Obote regime had become very tense, and freedom of speech was more controlled than ever before. Political comments could easily "result into death penalty or torture and incarceration."[143] In their attempt to be careful, their performances became monotonous, and the group lost their audience, and with it went the motivation of its members. Interestingly, there seems to be a pronounced difference in what rural and urban audiences expect of a theatre performance. As Kaahwa points out, in her home district, the entertaining comedies of the urban areas are not popular at all, and people keep away from urban visiting groups. Some adults even discourage as many people as possible from attending the shows. Popular urban theatre groups are regarded as merely a "bunch of clowns."[144] Not surprisingly, therefore, the youth theatre group lost their audience when they limited their performances to music shows. By 1986, the group no longer existed. With the new political climate after the end of the liberation war, they reemerged and sang praise songs for the National Resistance Army Youths.[145] Today, *Crude Theatre* in their dramatic sketches deal with current issues, such as problems of politics and economics, of the mentally and physically handicapped, of prisoners and of the old people.[146]

---

[142] Jessica Kaahwa, "Beyond the Pleasure Principle: the Sociological Impetus on the Theatre in Uganda: A Case Study of Country Side Youth Crude Theatre of Kibingo-Village, Bughaya Subcounty, Hoima District," unpublished paper at the Department of Music, Dance and Drama, Makerere University, Kampala, Uganda, 1990.

[143] ibid., p. 3.

[144] ibid., p. 1.

[145] Many of the NRA's members who fought in the bush with Yoweri Museveni, were teenage-soldiers of about fifteen to seventeen years of age.

[146] Jessica Kaahwa initiated the term *Crude Theatre*, with permission from the group, to define their format of presentation, including "the actors actions on stage, the staging, and the general structure in which they perform, the language, the seating facility."

In their attempt to discuss topical social problems, the group developed a play about AIDS. The action tells the story of a young girl in the village who is forced by her parents to marry a man much older than herself. Although she is in love with someone else, she follows her parents' order and marries the old man. The marriage, however, is not happy. Eventually, she leaves her husband and runs off to the city. There, she becomes a prostitute and dies of AIDS. Although for the spectator the impression may arise that the play argues against traditional values such as obedience towards elders, Jessica Kaahwa claims that the group is not at all against the observation of cultural norms. What they oppose is rather the rigid attitude of some people towards those norms. *Crude Theatre* advocate an adaptation of traditional laws to present-day life.

The group thinks theatre should be used for problem solving. They even set an example within their own group. One of their members is an ex-convict whom they accepted as a member, and who proved to be very talented. He thus had a chance to escape the vicious circle of criminality and start a new life. Kanyuyuzi, the leader of the group, relates the boy's development:

> That boy (Bingi) you see, is an exconvict, disowned by his family and an outcast of the village. But since he joined our group, Bingi has not only proved talented but very determined to prove people wrong of their notions about exconvicts. Bingi's case is a puzzle to all of us and the entire village. His talent for stringed instruments is boundless. But before we could get him to join the Youth group, Bingi was on verge of committing suicide out of dejection. I am happy to say that the boy has gained his old self and he feels himself existing.[147]

One of *Crude Theatre's* goals for the future is to get the authorization to perform in prisons out of a belief that "the exercise for humanizing" should start there.[148] Once the convicts are released, they are more ready to look at the world outside positively.

The commitment to involve prisoners in their theatre work points to the fact that *Crude Theatre* encourages all members of the community to participate and develop their creative talents. Theatre for them serves a cathartic purpose. During some shows, for example, they employ a traditional form of oral recitation and encourage the old ones among the spectators to relate stories from their youth and thus involve them in their

147 Kaahwa, "Beyond the Pleasure Principle," p. 7.

148 ibid., p. 10.

plays. This has the effect of helping them to "build a stronger self image."[149] Looking at the group's commitment for the people of Kibingo, it is not surprising that the community contributes to its existence with material and moral support: "Therefore, the popularity, the *Crude Theatre* is enjoying can be adduced to general response, altogether with the youth's format of getting all the people to participate in the construction of the structure and being present at the discussions that relate to the group, and sometimes do have open rehearsals. In this way people do identify with the group completely."[150]

The strong impact theatre may have on opinion-building can be seen in one of *Crude Theatre's* more politically oriented plays. In the performance, they discussed the issue of medical cost sharing which had been proposed by Government instead of free medical treatment. The debate was continued by the audience after the performance. In the play, on one side of the stage, a well equipped hospital is depicted. On the other side the poor masses die because they cannot pay for the expensive treatment. The climax of the play is a scene in which a doctor refuses to attend to a sick child whose mother has no money. Consequently the child dies, and the upset mother wails loudly in front of the clinic. As a crowd gathers, she narrates what has happened. The angry crowd storms the clinic, and the corrupt doctor has to escape through the window. The play ends with all the people helping the mother to carry her dead child, shouting slogans against cost sharing.[151] The production succeeded in increasing the people's awareness of the problem, and they started opposing it. The atmosphere became so tense that the farmers lost interest in their work and the crop harvest was affected. Eventually, "the bill was scraped before commencement."[152]

Crude Theatre's plans for the near future are to start open air performances to raise funds for the building of a theatre by the side of Lake Albert. Although the Kibingo villagers help the youths as well as they can, their financial situation is difficult. As Kaahwa remarks, *Crude Theatre* treats social issues in the community in a rather aggressive way.[153] She defines the groups' approach towards community life and ethics as being sociologically

---

[149] ibid., p. 11.

[150] ibid., p. 14.

[151] ibid., p. 17.

[152] Kaahwa, "Beyond the Pleasure Principle," p. 18.

[153] ibid., p. 18.

oriented rather than theatrically, concluding that the aim of *Crude Theatre* is to liberate the minds of the people from over-dependancy on the system. "In the process of liberation, self esteem is instilled in the people, thereby inspiring a patriotic spirit of service to the nation."[154]

2.3.1.4. Campaign Theatre

The activities of groups like *Crude Theatre* and comparatively small TFD projects carried out by NGOs should not give a wrong impression, however. Theatre for Development activities in Uganda during the last three to four years have mainly taken the form of nationwide information campaigns.[155] The plays do not, as is the case with rural TFD, have clear-cut target audiences, which are characterized by the area in which they live and by a common local problem which needs to be solved.[156] Target audiences for urban Campaign Theatre, which is concerned with health education, are not as well defined. They are spread all over the town, and they have to be seen in such categories as school-children, students, different professional groups etc. Unlike the projects by Muganga and Wadulo discussed above, Campaign Theatre which is concerned with topics such as AIDS education, can count on substantial financial resources provided by both GOs and NGOs. Especially NGOs and international organisations undertake to help Uganda in stopping the spread of the AIDS epidemic. An important step in this respect is the dissemination of information about the methods of transmission, prevention, condom use etc. This is done in large campaigns to reach as many people as possible. Breitinger draws attention to the fact that with this kind of theatre, a considerable part of the funding goes into the organisational set up rather than in the production of the shows, "with the risk that the funds might be diverted on the higher level of the campaign management."[157] Besides, since GOs, NGOs and international organisations are involved at the top of health education, they bring their own organisational pressures into the campaigns, since their officials are held responsible by the ministers or the chairmen of the organisation to prove results. Those results, however, are not necessarily measured according to medical or theatrical, but according to administrative, or

[154] ibid., p. 18.

[155] for definition of the term 'Campaign Theatre,' s. Introduction.

[156] Breitinger, "Popular Urban Theatre," p. 283.

[157] ibid, p. 287.

political criteria.[158] Immediate results measured in quantifyable data, e.g. the number of performances, number of spectators, number of participants etc. have to be achieved. As Breitinger further observes, this inevitably gives rise to big events, like festivals, because they attract maximum media coverage. Since the AIDS education campaign in Uganda focusses strongly on young people, i.e. school children who are not yet infected with the disease, Byron Kawadwa's idea of school drama competitions has been taken up again.

One such nationwide school drama competition was held as early as 1988. Among the prize-winning plays was *The Six Killer Diseases*, performed by the City Primary School of Kampala. The play follows the model of the biblical allegory. The six killer diseases - whooping cough, measles, diarrhoea, diphteria, small pox and cholera - together with their new brother AIDS, appear personified on stage, as the Seven Deadly Sins, acting "like 'old vices,' the villainous protagonists of the early Elizabethan and late medieval theatrical convention."[159] The diseases hold a meeting where they discuss their future plan of action. In the face of immunization campaigns by doctors, health officers and organisations like UNICEF, their 'work' has been rendered less and less effective. They complain that all of them will disappear if health education is taken seriously and everybody is immunised. Most of the communication is done verbally with each of the diseases giving a report. Otherwise, there is hardly any acting on stage. After a while, AIDS joins them declaring that if they cannot kill anymore, he will take over and kill on their behalf. Unlike the other killer diseases who were presented with some humour, in the case of Mr. AIDS it is communicated clearly that he is a lethal threat. With its ironical inversion of moral values the play is adapted to the juvenile psyche, but it is the form of the personal testimonial that carries dramatic conviction.[160]

After that festival, emphasis in Campaign Theatre was laid even more on AIDS education. The reason for this is twofold. On the one hand, the seriousness of the HIV/AIDS epidemic makes information campaigns necessary. On the other, there is a huge amount of donor money made available for educational campaigns. In 1989, there was the AIDS Quake Festival, jointly organised by the World Health Organization (WHO), the

---

[158] ibid., p. 287.

[159] ibid., p. 283.

[160] for further details about *The Six Killer Diseases*, s. Breitinger, "Popular Urban Theatre."

Global Programme on AIDS (GPA) and the Association of Performing Artists in Uganda (APAU).[161] Two years later, in 1991, another school drama competition was held, organised by UNICEF. This time, one play, *The Riddle*, containing all the information about AIDS, was to be performed by all primary schools in the country. The aim was that by acting out the AIDS information, the pupils would internalise the message and also spread it at home and among their friends.[162]

The survey of TFD activities given here tried to describe the historical and political context in which Theatre for Development in Uganda takes place. It showed that TFD, with the exception of *Crude Theatre*, does not try to influence the political situation in the country directly. Instead, the plays are informative, trying to educate the population about development aims. This approach stands in contrast to TFD plays in other African countries, as described in 2.1. A comparison of the political situation before and after 1986 explains that difference. When regarding TFD in Uganda today, one has to take into account the evolutionary development that theatre in general has experienced during the political turmoil of the last 20 years. Moreover, the current problems society in post-civil war Uganda is facing have to be considered. After 20 years of civil war, the economy is at its lowest point, and the country has to solve problems such as underdevelopment due to ignorance in the rural areas, a high occurence of diseases, infrastructural development and the AIDS-epidemic.

TFD is not politically committed in that it does not criticise the Government. Unlike many of the plays in other countries, it is not revolutionary. Nevertheless, it aims at positive social change by creating an awareness in the people of their own ability to act. TFD projects require funding, which in Uganda comes either from Government, or from NGOs and international organisations who work in collaboration with the Government. Topics that are discussed in TFD-plays such as AIDS, malnutrition of children, immunization etc. are issues that cause world-wide concern and maximum media coverage. International organisations like UNICEF, Red Cross, and WHO, therefore come and provide funding to help in the solution of those problems. Obviously, projects that are financed like that, do not criticise the Government's political actions. TFD in Uganda indeed is politically committed: it supports the Government's development

[161] for a detailed discussion, s. chapter 4.2.1.

[162] for a detailed discussion, s. chapter 4.2.2.

activities, i.e. Theatre for Development in Uganda has become a governmental instrument for change.

In the years between the 1950s and 70s, the various theatre groups catered for their respective expatriate, African, Indian or Goan audiences. This division no longer holds true in post-civil war Uganda. Theatrical groups still have different target audiences for their productions in mind, but the definition of those target audiences is now done according to social/economic rather than ethnic criteria. The aim of the production, i.e. information/education or entertainment, defines the target audience. TFD plays about health education therefore are designed for those social groups who are most likely to be affected by health risks. Plays for AIDS information for example are performed for target audiences such as schoolchildren, students and different professional groups. Popular urban comedies also have their specific audiences. The audience who goes to see a group like JK Ebonita at the Theatre Excelsior, typically includes newly-rich business men, merchants, traders, ex-patriates, etc., whereas the spectators of plays performed in backyards of pubs, by groups like the Bamazinga Dramatic Society, live in the slum areas of Kampala. Virtually all theatre groups in Uganda today have in common that they are non-professional, i.e. their members work as civil servants, office clerks, teachers, during the day and just come for rehearsals and performances in the evenings and on weekends. It is, therefore, a welcome addition to their low salaries when international organisations and NGOs employ them in the service of their information campaigns. This strategy of NGOs is typical for CT and will be discussed in more detail in the following chapter.

The influence of the literary dramatists of the 1960s and 70s on present-day TFD, therefore, is more of an indirect nature. Due to the civil war, there was no uninterrupted development of Ugandan Theatre between 1968 and 1986. A result is that we have the literary dramatists of the 60s and 70s on one side, and present-day TFD and comedies on the other. The impact of the playwrights Serumaga, Ssentongo, Kawadwa et al. on modern productions can still be traced, however. Even though Serumaga's plays have not been performed since the late 1960s, they are available as playscripts, and many playwrights and actors still remember them. Byron Kawadwa's *Song of Wankoko* is still performed today in front of sold out houses. With his play, Kawadwa had succeeded in "creating a model which many aspiring young dramatists tried to follow."[163] The plays of all three authors, Serumaga, Ssentongo, and Kawadwa are on the syllabus of the Department for Music, Dance and Drama at Makerere University - through which many of the influential theatre practitioners have gone before they joined popular urban groups like Ebonita or took up work with GOs and NGOs to produce didactic plays. In the analysis of the case studies, I will show what kind of dramatic techniques today's playwrights took from the literary dramatists. Secondly, by demonstrating how the modern playwrights changed and adapted those techniques to present-day conditions, the influence of politics on theatre in the specific Ugandan context will become obvious.

Before going on to describe concrete examples of TFD as it is practiced in Uganda, some theoretical considerations will have to be taken into account. In connection with health-related topics, certain organisational structures in TFD have emerged that can best be described with the term 'Campaign Theatre' (CT): theatre is used by Western NGOs and international organisations in the service of their information campaigns. In order to communicate effectively, the plays not only have to consider the country's political and social history. Their forms, techniques and content also have to be in accordance with the culture and its norms and values. This is not always easy since CT as a form of communication for mass mobilization usually involves members of different cultures. In the following chapter, mechanisms and context of this type of theatre will be described and theoretical principles, such as forms and techniques will be analysed. Since CT is a comparatively new phenomenon, a systematic theory of it does not exist. In order to describe it adequately, I found it useful to combine various theoretical approaches; consequently, findings of general communication theory will be combined with those of intercultural communication theory and semiotics of culture, and later related to CT as it is performed in Uganda.

---

163 Breitinger, "Popular Urban Theatre," p. 271.

3. CAMPAIGN THEATRE - A THEORETICAL APPROACH

3.1. Semiotics of Culture

In order to fully understand the way communication works between participants in the communication process of Campaign Theatre, a digression into the semiotics of culture is helpful. This will shed light on the various reasons for misunderstandings in the communication between the cultures. By including a chapter on various social and ethic concepts of Ganda society, I will demonstrate how misunderstandings occur and how they can be avoided in the particular Ugandan context.

Semiotics of culture can only be meaningfully discussed within the context of modern semiotics in general. As Thomas Winner in "Some Fundamental Concepts Leading to a Semiotics of Culture" points out, questions relating to the interdependence of semiotic systems in general and particularly questions concerning the relation of natural language as the privileged sign system[1] to other systems were hardly addressed in a systematic way during the two thousand years of the history of semiotics.[2] It was not until the late 1920s and early 1930s that "the first steps were taken to lay the groundwork for modern semiotic theory in general, and for a theory of semiotics of culture in particular."[3] In 1926, a group of Russian and Czech scholars formed the Prague Linguistic Circle. Their work not only influenced structural linguistics and the study of natural language as a sign system, but also the semiotics of other systems and a theory of the interrelationship between the systems.[4] When regarding CT from the viewpoint of a semiotics of culture, the relevance of their findings is evident. In the following, I will briefly outline their most influential theories. This will both place the theoretical approach I take in this chapter in its historical context, as well as explain its relevance to Campaign Theatre.

---

1 The term 'natural language' is used to distinguish spoken/written languages, such as e.g. English, French etc., from other sign systems, such as dress, arts etc., which also function as languages.

2 Thomas Winner, "Some Fundamental Concepts Leading to a Semiotics of Culture: A Historical Overview," in *Semiotics of Culture*, ed. Irene Portis Winner and Jean Umiker Sebeok (The Hague, Paris, New York: Mouton Publishers, 1979).

3 Winner, "Some Fundamental Concepts," p. 75.

4 ibid, p. 75.

The contribution of the Prague Linguistic Circle to a later theory of semiotics of culture was essentially in three areas: a) the position that sign systems are not totally immanent, i.e. that they are interrelated to other systems which exist independently outside of them; b) the view of function and of the polyfunctional nature of human activity; c) the view of the existence of other sign-systems, apart from natural language, which form a complex system of semiotic codes: arts, codes of dress, various ethnographic information systems etc.[5] One of their most significant contributions to the semiotics of culture is the discussion of the immanence of structures. The work of art is seen by the Prague Linguistic Circle as autonomous, because it is organised according to its own structural rules and evolves according to these. It also exists in complex relations to other structures such as society, or the author's or reader's psyche. Those relationships need to be taken into account, especially when examining the evolution of artistic forms.[6] All cultural phenomena were regarded as mutually interdependent. Language was considered the key to the articulation of the work of art with extra-literary systems. Language in its turn, is linked to the value systems of a culture in a given period. The view of the complexity of the relations of language to literature and structures external to it, as advanced by Jan Mukarovsky, one of the leading figures of the Prague Linguistic Circle, anticipates "the contemporary position that culture may be understood as a complex semiotic system of information, which is advanced by the Tartu-Moscow scholars and others."[7]

The most important contribution of the Prague group of linguists to the semiotics of culture, is its extension of semiotics from natural language to other cultural systems. The discussions and views of the Prague group about such issues as the question and meaning of art, the relation of a work of art to its creator and the perceivers, the complex interrelationship between art, culture and society, the relationships of different arts to each other, and the evolution of artistic systems - laid the foundation for modern semiotics. They influenced the Tartu-Moscow school of semiotics, the Polish and Czeck schools, and also the semiotics of Western Europe, the Western Hemisphere, and Israel.[8]

---

5 ibid., p. 76.

6 ibid., p. 76.

7 ibid., p. 78.

8 ibid., p. 78/9.

The work of the Prague Linguistic Circle is relevant for a discussion of Campaign Theatre, because it shaped notions of contemporary semiotics of culture, such as the interrelatedness of systems, the polyfunctionality of human behaviour, and the opposition of the inner versus outer sphere of culture.[9] Those notions, in turn, are helpful when trying to understand the mechanisms of CT. In a programmatic statement, *Theses on the Semiotic Study of Culture* (1973), the basic assumption of cultural semiotics is that all human activity is concerned with the processing, exchange and storage of information:[10] "Thus culture is understood as a process and a mechanism characterized by the struggle for information which is received, accumulated, preserved, and coded, decoded and translated from one system into another, as well as exchanged."[11]

In the following, those findings of contemporary semiotics of culture relevant to an explanation of the communication process through TFD will be discussed. For that purpose, I refer to works that concern themselves directly with intercultural communication rather than with a theory of communication in general.[12]

3.2. Culture - Development - Communication

After almost four decades of development policies, we now realise that earlier models for development were inadequate. Prior policies were based on a linear view of progress which assumed economic growth would automatically trigger socio-cultural changes. More recently, the question has been asked what actually defines a development goal. The realization has

---

9 s. chapter 3.7.

10 *Theses on the Semiotic Study of Culture*, 1973 drawn up by five Russian scholars: B.A. Uspenskij, V.V. Ivanov, V.N. Toporov, A.M. Pjatigorskij, J.M. Lotman; for discussion of the *Theses* s. Irene Portis Winner and Thomas Winner, "The Semiotics of Cultural Texts," in *Semiotica, 18:2* (The Hague, Paris: Mouton Publishers, 1976); and I. Winner, "Ethnicity, Modernity, and Theory of Culture Texts," in *Semiotics of Culture*, p. 106/7.

11 I. Winner, "Ethnicity, Modernity, and Theory of Culture Texts," p. 106/7.

12 Semiotic works by scholars like Kristeva, Deleuze and Guattari, Lotman, Derrida, Uspenskij, and the discussion of their findings in articles by I. Winner, T. Winner, Grossberg, Culler, Rewar et al. I found helpful, but not directly relating to the phenomenon of CT; for a more detailed discussion of the theory of semiotics of culture s. I. Winner, "Ethnicity, Modernity, and Theory of Culture Texts." In *Semiotics of Culture*; T. Winner, "Some Fundamental Concepts Leading to a Semiotics of Culture"; Julia Kristeva, *Die Revolution der poetischen Sprache*; Roman Jakobson, *Aufsätze zur Linguistik und Poetik*; Eco, *Einführung in die Semiotik*; Mukarovsky, *Kapitel aus der Ästhetik*; Lotman, *Die Struktur literarischer Texte*; et al.

come that the growth of the gross national product is not necessarily a valid measure of human well-being and the quality of life. As Janusz Ziolkowski correctly points out, any kind of development goal necessarily becomes a socio-cultural goal, because it affects at least a portion of society. Resolution No. 2626 (XXV) on International Development Strategy for the Second United Nations Development Decade states that "qualitative and structural changes in society must go hand in hand with rapid economic growth, and existing disparities - regional, sectoral and social - should be substantially reduced. These objectives are both determining factors and end-results of development."[13] That statement takes the fact into account that development, even if it is gradual, means a social transformation, a transformation of identity, the end point being very different from the starting point. Values, aspirations, aims, convictions cannot "provide the value premises which would justify the terminal condition."[14] Besides, the resolution regards man not as an object, resource, or capital. It considers man as an end of all economic activity.[15]

We now recognise that development is a complex, multidimensional process whose single aspects cannot be regarded in isolation. An integrated approach to development is necessary, one which takes account of those interdependencies: "The integrated conduct of development should be a means of directing it towards the attainment of far-reaching and freely accepted ends - necessarily socio-cultural in character; integration implies interdisciplinary reflection, stock-taking and a return to origins, i.e. the culture of a given society."[16] Communication between the target group and those who want to implement a development programme in this respect plays a vital role. Since development projects most often are financed and partly organised by non-indigenous organisations who do not come from the same culture as the target group, the communication between the members of the different cultures poses a problem. In order to ensure the success of the intercultural communication, an awareness of different thought concepts in the cultures between the communicators is therefore necessary.

---

13 Para. 18 of Resolution No. 2626 (XXV) on International Development Strategy for the Second United Nations Development Decade; also quoted in Janusz Ziolkowsky, "Cultural Dimension of Development," in *Cultures*, Vol. VI, no. 1. (Paris: the Unesco Press and la Baconnière, 1979)

14 Ziolkowski, "Cultural Dimension of Development," p. 18.

15 ibid.

16 ibid., p. 19.

Every communication system has a sender and a receiver. The sender produces patterns of behaviour or 'qualities of expression' that express attitudes towards the world. The receiver obtains a message through the interpretation of those patterns of behaviour. The patterns of behaviour and 'qualities of expression' come into existence through signals, signs and symbols which carry meaning.[17] Meaning, however, can only be constituted if there exists a code which is used by both sender and recipient. The description of symbols is difficult, since their meaning depends entirely on cultural agreements, which function according to a system of rules only known to its users.[18] According to Victor Turner, three dimensions have to be considered when trying to understand the meaning of a symbol:[19] the *exegetic* dimension which contains the complete set of explanations for a given symbol - a dimension which is only known by the users; the *operational* dimension which equates the meaning of a symbol with its use; and the *positional* dimension according to which the meaning of a symbol depends on its relation to other symbols.[20] The different attitudes occurring in intercultural communication are expressed through codes, and so not surprisingly, in a conference on intercultural communication theory (1983), the importance of codes in communication was particularly stressed by dedicating one of the work-groups to it.[21] The discussion in the group was based on the definition of code as a "culturally defined, rule-governed system of shared arbitrary symbols used to transmit (and elicit) meaning. Included within the concept of code are language, paralinguistic phenomena, nonverbal phenomena, silence, language choice, multilingual

---

17 Edmund Leach, *Kultur und Kommunikation. Zur Logik symbolischer Zusammenhänge*, p. 17; Mario von Cranach, "Die nichtverbale Kommunikation im Kontext des kommunikativen Verhaltens," p. 126; Arnold Niederer, "Zur Ethnographie und Soziographie nicht-verbaler Dimensionen der Kommunikation," p. 1; quoted in Jutta Weidig, *Tanz-Ethnologie. Einführung in die völkerkundliche Sicht des Tanzes* (Ahrensburg bei Hamburg: Verlag Ingrid Czwalina, 1984), p. 68.

18 Weidig, *Tanz-Ethnologie*, p. 68.

19 Victor Turner, "Forms of Symbolic Action: Introduction," in R.F. Spencer, ed., *Forms of Symbolic Action. Proceedings of the 1969 Annual Spring Meeting of the American Ethnological Society* (Seattle, London, 1969), pp. 3-25.

20 ibid., p. 68.

21 Action Caucus and Seminar on Theory in Intercultural Communication, described by L.E. Sarbaugh and Nobleza Asuncion-Lande, "Theory Building in Intercultural Communication: Synthesizing the Action Caucus," in *Intercultural Communication Theory. Current Perspectives*, ed. W. Gudykunst (Beverly Hills, London, New Delhi: Sage Publications, 1984).

behaviour, interruptions, turn-taking, and organisation of talk."[22] The work group argued for a set of principles which would help organise contexts according to the place in a society's organisation of its everyday world. This could be done through ethnographic analysis of the communication process in a community that would take account of the interdependence between code, culture and communication. The importance of this relationship came up again in the report of one of the other work-groups, the 'constructivism' group, which recognised the extent to which the culture and the social world into which one is born influence the cognitive themes by which one interprets the world. Representatives of 'ethnoscience' which is concerned with how different ethnic groups classify objects of their world or aspects of their culture, share this opinion: the conceptual system of each people is unique and can only be understod within its own conditions ("die Begriffswelt eines jeden Volkes ist einzigartig und kann nur mit ihren eigenen Bedingungen verstanden werden").[23]

TFD tries to overcome those barriers in intercultural communication. By involving the target group, the need to include its culture into the development process is met, and self-awareness is brought to its members. Owing to the direct interaction between communicators and target group, TFD is more and more appreciated as an instrument for communication. It offers a clear advantage over the mass media, where direct interaction is not possible, thereby neglecting "what seems to be the critical functions of communication in the processes of mdernization and social change, i.e. the epistemic differentiation and pluralization of life worlds and the need for more rational and humane systems of knowledge, organisation, and reconciliation of the conflicting sources of identity, authority, and legitimacy."[24] As Majid Tehranian correctly states, mass media by definition treat their audiences as homogeneous and undifferentiated. They impose their message on the audience and leave no room for immediate response. Communication through mass media therefore is no longer a two-way process. Tehranian even goes so far as to say they produce alienation and protest in those countries in which the growth of mass communication has outpaced literacy. Mass media do not leave any room for the development

22 ibid., p. 48.

23 Roger Keesing, *Cultural Anthropology. A Contemporary Perspective*," p. 173, transl. by Weidig, *Tanz-Ethnologie*, p. 69; s.a. Sturtevant, "Studies in Ethnoscience," p. 99.

24 Majid Tehranian, "Communication and Intercultural Development: Some Theoretical Considerations," in *Cultures*, Vol. VI, 1979, p. 31

of voluntary associations and the possibilities for cognitive participation. They tend to be used by the ruling groups for cognitive domination.[25] The Brasilian Paulo Freire also draws attention to the well-known fact that when people are denied their right to participate in history as subjects that they become dominated and alienated.[26] In his model of education he particularly stresses the need for dialogue as opposed to what he calls the 'banking concept' by which he means an education which has become an act of depositing, in which the students are the depositories, and the teacher is the depositor. Instead of communicating, the teacher issues communiqués which are quietly received by the students.[27] Freire argues for a liberated education instead, that consists in acts of cognition rather than pure transferrals of information. What he demands with regard to education, particularly adult education, also applies to development projects. More often than not, they are brought into the communities from outside, whereas it should be the communities who articulate their ideas about development. It has been realised, however, that the 'banking concept' - in form of western development planners deciding what is needed in the so-called Third World Countries, implementing it and teaching the population how to use it - is no longer possible. What is needed is a concept of development that comes from within the target group and takes into account its culture. TFD does that by involving both the target group and its culture, as well as, by its very nature, making dialogue possible between communicators and audience.

3.3. The Communication Process

In his article, "Adaptive Intercultural Communication," Huber Ellingsworth describes intercultural communication.[28] He divides the communication process as it occurs in interpersonal communication into sub-units such as 'participants,' 'setting,' 'purpose,' 'process' and 'outcome.' Those parameters can also be employed for a detailed description of the communication process in TFD plays. In order to clarify some aspects of CT on which I will

---

25 ibid., p. 31.

26 Paulo Freire, *Pedagogy of the Oppressed* (Suffolk: Penguin Books, 1972), p. 101.

27 ibid., p. 45 ff.

28 Huber W. Ellingsworth, "Adaptive Intercultural Communication," in *Intercultural Communiction Theory. Current Perspectives*, ed. W. Gudykunst (Beverly Hills, London, New Delhi: Sage Publications, 1984).

focus later on in the discussion, I will at this point briefly present the parameters according to Ellingsworth's division.

3.3.1. Participants

Communication takes place between participants. In the case of TFD, the participants are the sponsors of the play, the playwrights, the actors on stage and the audience. The communication qualifies as intercultural since its participants belong to different cultures. Most of the TFD plays in Uganda concerned with AIDS-information are financed by international organisations or NGOs whose members usually come from Europe or the U.S. In all likelihood, the audience itself comprises members of different ethnic groups, especially in a city like Kampala. Therefore, a possibility of misunderstanding and disagreement arising from different belief and value systems of the participants exists. If successful communication is to occur, the similarities and differences between the participants have to be acknowledged.[29]

3.3.2. Setting

The communication takes place in a particular setting. Ellingsworth suggests an ideal setting in a neutral place where all participants can meet on equal terms, without role differences and power inequity. He admits, however, that most communications occur at settings that contribute to the inequality between the participants. A TFD play performed at a theatre hall is less likely to effect successful communication than a performance outside in the round. The proscenium-stage usually found in theatre halls creates an inequality between spectators and actors that discourages audience participation.[30]

3.3.3. Process

The process of intercultural communication concerns adaptation. Ellingsworth identifies the use of communicative strategies growing out of congruence of purpose as another dynamic dimension - which is the case in Ugandan TFD that is concerned with AIDS: all participants - sponsors,

29 ibid., p. 198; s.a. chapter 3.7.

30 The factor 'setting' will be discussed in more detail in chapter 4.1.

playwrights, actors, audience - want to fight AIDS. When the participants agree that their interests are mutual, cooperative strategies of adaptation will appear, so that differences in belief and value system can be compensated. All participants of the strategy share the wish to stop the growth of the AIDS epidemic. Accordingly, they make efforts to reach an understanding.

3.3.4. Outcome

For interpersonal communication, Ellingsworth distinguishes between purposeful and personal outcomes. Some outcomes are related to the achievement, modification, or thwarting of the original purposes, and some to the effect of the communication on the participants. Ellingsworth advocates mutual adaptation of all participants, so that intercultural communication can occur. Transferred to TFD, the most important criterion when judging the outcome is whether the message of the play has convinced the audience to change their behaviour or not. Obviously, this applies to intercultural communication as well as to communication in general. The dialogue between participants can then result in an alteration of the individual's culture-based beliefs.[31]

3.4. Barriers to effective communication

Since communication through TFD most often is intercultural, more has to be said about misunderstandings, and how they occur in intercultural communication.

In order to explain the phenomenon, Peter Ehrenhaus convincingly applies Fritz Heider's attribution theory.[32] Attribution theory is concerned with the manner in which people organise the stream of information received from the environment into meaningful events and actions. Heider regards the attribution process as a continuous stream rather than as a series of stages. The process usually happens automatically when attributors approach interactions with expectations which make it possible to assign significance to experience and interaction. Most often, we perceive and

---

31 Ellingsworth, "Adaptive Intercultural Communication," p. 203.

32 Peter Ehrenhaus, "Culture and the Attribution Process: Barriers to Effective Communication," in *Intercultural Communication Theory. Current Perspectives*, ed. W. Gudykunst (Beverly Hills, London, New Delhi: Sage Publications, 1984), p. 259 ff.

comprehend at the same time when structures of expectations guide us to organise actions into meaningful units. These structures are influenced by the attributor's culture: "These conceptual structures are inductively derived and probalistic and they are based upon our experiences of the world within some culture or series of cultures."[33] Ehrenhaus poses the hypothesis that in initial intercultural interactions, communicators will seek out information deemed salient by everybody. This decision, however, is based on presuppositions of their respective cultures - which will be the source of misattributions about each other.[34] A number of studies have revealed that what is judged to be salient depends on the individuum's belonging to either High Context Culture (HCC) or Low Context Culture (LCC).[35] In HCCs, the information that is estimated as salient for learning about one another and to predict a person's behaviour is based on social background. The Ganda society would, according to this definition, be a HCC society. As in many other African societies, the welfare of the community is placed above that of the individuum. Western cultures on the other hand, with the central position they attribute to the individuum, tend to be LCC. These differences have to be taken into account when trying to communicate effectively between the cultures. Obviously, a high degree of attributional sensitivity is required. This also becomes evident when looking at Ehrenhaus' second hypothesis, i.e. that intercultural communicators are particularly likely to commit the "ultimate attribution error."[36] He draws attention to some findings of attribution research which have shown that contextual and social constraints upon actors are usually underestimated, whereas personal dispositions are overestimated. The "ultimate attribution error" is at its most extreme when people are prejudiced.[37]

In order to avoid cultural misunderstandings, Paulo Freire stresses the need for thorough thematic investigation before trying to inform and educate a community. The investigation has to be done together with the members of the community, thereby becoming a "common striving towards

33 ibid., p. 262.

34 ibid., p. 264.

35 High Context Culture: communicative behaviour is to a higher proportion a product of situational forces rather than of the internal characteristics of the interactants; Low Context Culture: relatively little information about physical or social context to guide the attribution process is available; s. Ehrenhaus, "Culture and the Attribution Process," p. 263.

36 ibid., p. 266.

37 Pettigrew in Ehrenhaus, "Culture and the Attribution Process," p. 266.

awareness of reality and self, thus making it a starting point for the educational process or for cultural action of a liberating character."[38] Thematic investigation thus becomes a process of search, of knowledge, and eventually of creation. Freire also draws attention to the fact that this process must include a concern for the links between the themes as well as a concern for their historical-cultural context. Investigation has to be done, therefore, into people's thinking, so they can produce and act upon their own ideas instead of absorbing those of others.

TFD with its characteristic involvement of the target community in the project, seems particularly well-suited as a means of information and education according to Freire's demands. Before discussing the social and cultural context of TFD in Uganda, I would like to present some thoughts about theatre as a medium for didactic messages in general. A look at certain characteristics inherent in the medium theatre as well as at its historical context in Africa, explains why theatre plays an important part in the search for new means of disseminating information on the side of GOs, NGOs and IOs. In their search for new channels of information which involves the target communities as more equal partners in the process, rather than just as a passive audience, they increasingly rely on theatre.

3.5. Theatre as a Medium

Theatre as a basic medium is well-suited for mass mobilisation. Leonard Doob distinguishes two kinds of media, i.e basic and extending media. The distinction is based on the position of the communicator in relation to the audience: media where a communicator is physically present are defined as basic media.[39] Those media, on the other hand, that do not require the presence of the communicator, are extending media. TFD, therefore, in its original sense, is a basic medium: a message is conveyed from the actors on stage to the audience. Especially with regard to TFD in Uganda it is evident that the actors often are not the original communicators. What we have, is a chain of communicators ranging from personnel in international organisations who brief artists; who in turn create plays which eventually are performed by the actors.[40] In some cases, TFD may even fall under the

38 Freire, *Pedagogy of the Oppressed*, p. 79.

39 Leonard W. Doob, *Communication in Africa. A Search for Boundaries* (Westport, Connecticut: Greenwood Press, Publishers, 1961), p. 57.

40 for a detailed discussion s. chapter 3.8.

category 'extending media': when TFD plays are recorded on video, as was the case with the non-Government organisation *The Experiment in International Living* (EIL) and their play *It's Not Easy*, which was then shown on information tours up-country.[41] It is obvious that the communicator in this case is not present. It is this characteristic of theatre as basic media that makes it particularly appropriate as a medium for mass mobilisation. The direct interaction between actors on stage and the audience creates a more personal atmosphere than video shows or newspaper texts.[42] Besides, the physical presence of the audience makes it possible to direct its attention to certain problems, and then re-enforce the information through discussions after the performance. Theatre is one of the few media where 'talking back' in form of questions, comments, and discussions is actually possible.

In Uganda, drama with its own characteristics seems to work very well as a channel to disseminate information. I partly agree with Doob when he defines drama as "the reproduction of fiction by one or more actors whose total behaviour resembles the behaviour of the real or imaginary characters in some type of setting."[43] As such, drama serves an emotive function and is able to convey information. While it is doubtlessly true that theatre works on an emotional level and thus is able to change behaviour, Doob's definition does not consider some other basic traits of theatre. Besides appealing to the audience's emotions, plays that try to raise consciousness also give factual information which refers to the rational part of the consciousness. It should also be noted that theatre is not merely the "reproduction of fiction," i.e. the performance of a written text. Even in literary drama/theatre, where we have an elaborated script, the performance is not merely an enactment of the written text. By transferring the message from the medium of written fiction to that of a life performance, it changes into something distinctly different. Theatre is a medium of its own with certain characteristics, that render it particularly suitable for communication of a didactic nature - in fact, more so than fiction. This becomes obvious when looking at the findings of one school of thought in communication theory, the technological determinist school,

---

41 s. chapter 4.4.1.

42 In the case of CT, however, it is important that the message reaches as many people as possible. From a logistical and financial stand-point, it is not practical to have troupes of actors going throughout the communities. It is more cost-effective to take pre-recorded tapes and show them to the audience; there should be time for questions and discussion afterwards; (conversations with L.B. Wilson, WHO).

43 Doob, *Communication in Africa*, p. 77.

which argues that the medium used to convey a message is of primary importance. Innis, an advocate of that school, states that any given medium will bias social organisation. He explains that time and space have taken on different cultural meanings - time meaning the sacred, the moral emphasis upon religion and hierarchy, and space the emphasis upon state, technical and secular development. That bias of media in favour of one institution also implies the assurance of cultural characteristics of that institution. As an example Mowlana gives the contrast between oral and written traditions: "Whereas oral culture tended to be time-binding with limited capacity for technical change, written tradition led to space-binding and consequently favored the growth of political authority."[44] One of the most pronounced adherents of that school of thought, Marshall McLuhan, even goes so far as to say that the medium itself is the message: "The things on which words were written down count more than the words themselves."[45] In contrast to Innis who thinks that the medium of communication affects social organisation, McLuhan finds its effect to be on sensory organisation and thought. His hypothesis is that the West has lost its balance because with print and writing it allowed sight to take precedence over other senses. Peoples belonging to oral cultures on the other hand, who prefer speech to writing, by using their sensoriae, live in a more vivid world and therefore are in balance with their environment.[46] As Mowlana correctly argues, the technological determinist school of thought focusses too narowly on only one aspect of communication, the technological one. Besides, the approach is based on Western experience and on the historical evidence with no dynamism of its own.[47] Nevertheless, the approach is interesting because it puts so much stress on the importance of the medium. Especially McLuhan's argument that written tradition neglects the other senses seems to speak in favour of TFD as a medium for communication. In theatre, sensations are stirred not only by the visual sense, but also by such parameters as sound, rhythm, words. Besides, participation of the audience is possible. Doob makes the point that theatre as a medium appeals most instantly to many African societies, because most of them have a long

---

44 Hamid Mowlana, "Mass Media and Culture: Toward an Integrated Theory," in *Intercultural Communication Theory. Current Perspectives*, ed. W. Gudykunst (Beverly Hills, London, New Delhi: Sage Publications, 1984), p. 153.

45 McLuhan, cited in Mowlana, "Mass Media and Culture," p. 153.

46 ibid., p. 153.

47 ibid., p. 154.

theatre tradition.[48] For Uganda, this is only partly true. Theatre, as we understand it today, was unknown until its introduction by the colonialists. Rather than theatre, story-telling as a dramatic genre of narration has been used to pass on knowledge and to comment on society.[49] Accordingly, Babacar Siné in his study on new communication techniques in black Africa demands a critical evaluation of the ancient methods of communication which Africa invented.[50] He draws attention to the fact that Africa has always "conversed and put questions within itself by means of communications adjusted to its own human dimensions, in the villages or in small animated communities; the transmitters were not anonymous and the "public," far from being a passive receiver and an impotent consumer, took part in a dialectic of communication based on dialogue and participation."[51] Those ancient means of communication contained the drum, the tam-tam, the palaver. To this list the theatre might be added. It is important to note that the audiences who received the messages took part in the communication process which was based on dialogue and participation. Hanna points out that education experts recommend in order to change opinions and attitudes, sensory experience should be as complete as possible.[52] In a theatre play, a variety of sensory stimuli are at work: movement, a kinesthetic activity or empathy, the sight of performers, sometimes the participation of the audience. In her analysis of how dance-plays operate, she draws attention to findings from psychology on how opinions and attitudes are changed. Accordingly, strong appeals are more effective than mild ones when communicated by credible sources; pleasant forms of distraction can increase the effectiveness of persuasive appeals; the impact of an appeal is enhanced by active audience participation, which also

---

48 Doob, *Communication in Africa*, p. 77.

49 It should be noted that drama in East Africa is a new form, although elements of it can be seen in traditional patterns of communication. The traditional story-teller for example told a story with many gestures and enactment of the dialogue. Elements of drama can also be seen in the traditional folk-songs and dances. As Margaret Macpherson concludes, however, none of these forms had taken the direction that would have produced the development of drama. When speaking of a traditional predisposition towards theatre as a means of communication therefore, I refer to elements of drama that existed in the traditional setting, rather than to the medium theatre as practised today.

50 Babacar Siné, "Cultural Dynamics and New Communication Techniques in Black Africa," in *Cultures*, Vol. VI, 1979, p. 74ff.

51 ibid., p. 75.

52 Judith Lynne Hanna, *To Dance is Human. A Theory of Nonverbal Communication* (Chicago and London: The University of Chicago press, 1987), p. 89

helps to overcome resistance to the message; repetition and active participation help to prevent the wearing off of a communication over time;[53] political perceptions develop and are reinforced and cognitions can be generated in large groups.[54] The conclusion Hanna draws for dance-plays also holds true for TFD: a performance can be "strong, pleasant, active, involving a repetitive appeal manipulated by a credible authority in a striking setting for a dramatically participating large public with a degree of consensus about shared meaning."[55] Maybe TFD with its encouragement of audience participation and discussion is a possibility to involve the traditional African characteristics of communication. Siné's criticism of the mass media superseding traditional communication systems brings TFD as an alternative to mind. He deplores the fact that media like radio, TV and cinema are "introduced in the form of a relay system whose objective is the cultural modelling of the "periphery" according to the canons and requirements of the "centre," which means an implacable extraversionist logic."[56] Siné sees as a reason for the fast spreading of mass media the audio-visual tradition already rooted in African societies. Oral expression is one of the major characteristics of that tradition "where pictures serve as existential support to artistic creativity and to daily communication."[57] This very disposition of African societies towards mass media in fact may also be favourable for the 'return' to a medium like theatre. It is able to refer to old structures of communication that are still familiar to the audiences, and as such it can be very effective.

Besides that traditional predisposition towards theatre as a channel of communication, in Uganda it is the only medium that is accessible to everybody. This becomes evident when one keeps in mind that 48% of the population is illiterate. TV can only be received in some areas in the south, and even there, most people cannot afford TV sets. Those who have one are subject to the all-too frequent power cuts, which makes television a comparatively unreliable instrument for the dissemination of any message. The same applies for radio. Since the power-situation is so unpredictable,

53 Marvin Karlins and Herbert Abelson, in Hanna, *To Dance is Human*, p. 90

54 Claus Mueller, in Hanna, *To Dance is Human*, p. 90.

55 ibid, p. 90.

56 ibid., p. 75.

57 ibid., p. 76/7

people have to use expensive batteries; not to speak of the costs for purchasing a radio.

Combining all the factors listed here, i.e. the story-telling-tradition, the need for entertainment as well as information, and the inaccessibility of all other media, theatre in the Ugandan context seems to be the most adequate way to reach as many people as possible. Besides, the speculation may hold true that, given the particular hierarchical structure of Ugandan society as will be described below, plays for consciousness raising with their asymetric form of communication, may work very well in the Ugandan context.[58]

3.6. Uganda in its Social Context

Representatives of all disciplines that concern themselves with communication (ethno-methodologists, sociolinguists, semioticians et al.) stress that communication is context bound and as such cannot be studied as isolated phenomenon.[59] Obviously, this also applies for communication through theatre. In plays dealing with AIDS information, concepts relating to Uganda's social framework are addressed. In all the plays, e.g., there are references to promiscuity as the cause for AIDS, and a monogamous life-style is suggested. In order to convince the audience, traditional moral values are alluded to. Other phenomena, like social structure, the effects of urbanisation on society as well as the attitude towards age and death, also play a role in the design of the plays. Therefore, before describing the actual phenomenon of CT, some of these concepts will have to be mentioned, so that the plays can be understood in their context.

3.6.1. Promiscuity

All plays about AIDS stress the fact the disease is transmitted through sexual intercourse and that the high promiscuity of society in Uganda has led to its rapid spread. The notion of promiscuity is expressed as being

---

58 I use the term 'asymetric communication' for plays which try to raise consciousness because they, unlike project-oriented plays, give information which does not come from within the target community and which is not disputable - although discussion between audience and communicators is still possible.

59 Ralph E. Cooley, "Codes and Contexts: An Argument For Their Description," in *Intercultural Communication Theory. Current Perspectives*, ed. W. Gudykunst (Beverly Hills, London, New Delhi: Sage Publications, 1984) p. 249; and Asuncion-Lande, Sarbaugh, p. 52, 48; s.a. view of the Prague School of Linguistics that all cultural phenomena are interrelated, chapter 3.1. of this study;

morally bad, and as a solution the plays suggest to adhere to principles like 'zero grazing' and 'love carefully.' It is made clear that promiscuity is a deviation from the established cultural or social values to which people should return. This European ethnocentric argument goes back to the days of the missionaries; the cultural stereotype of African promiscuity continues. It seems logical, therefore, that plays financed by international organisations suggest abandonment of promiscuity. The argument that the solution to conquer AIDS as suggested in the plays, is imposed upon the Ugandans by the members of international organisations is weakened, however, when one regards the workshop held for Ugandan artists before the AIDS Quake Festival.[60] In the workshop, which was organised by the World Health Organisation (WHO) and the Global Programme on AIDS (GPA), the artists were supposed to obtain the necessary information about the disease which they then could use to create educative plays. One important point for discussion was the transmission of AIDS. Besides sexual intercourse, other ways of infection were discussed, e.g. risk-enhancing cultural practices (circumcision, tatooes, etc.), blood transfusions, unclean needles etc. Interestingly, in the plays and songs the Ugandan artists created after the workshop, none of the concepts were depicted. They all concentrated on promiscuity as the cause for the spread of AIDS.[61]

In order to fully understand plays dealing with AIDS information, one has to keep in mind there are two different notions of promiscuity which should not be confused. One being the traditional Ugandan viewpoint, the other a Western perspective. Before colonialism, Ganda society used to have a very strict moral system with laws that had to be observed by everybody. Sexual relationships outside marriage were regarded as morally wrong. In a pamphlet on 'Education, Civilization and "Foreignization"', the *Kabaka* (King) deplores the disregard of that principle in modern Ganda society "although polygamy was universally recognised among the Baganda and was never considered as immoral yet prostitution was absolutely unheard of. Civilization, education and freedom are the direct causes of the appalling state of affairs as regards prostitution and promiscuous relationships between the Baganda men and women."[62] Joshua Sempebwa

60 for a detailed discussion of the workshop, s. the case studies in chapter 4.

61 for a detailed discussion of focus on promiscuity, s. chapter 3.6.1.

62 "Education, Civilization and "Foreignization" in Buganda." The Kabaka's pamphlet, 1935, printed in D.A. Low, *The Mind of Buganda. Documents of the Modern History of an African Kingdom* (London, Ibadan, Nairobi: Heinemann, 1971), p. 106.

explains that Ganda sexual morality can only be properly understood in terms of marriage which ensures lineage solidarity and fertility. The importance of fertility is strongly emphasized.[63] Adultery, in the Ugandan context, a man sleeping with a married woman, was strictly forbidden.[64] Whereas, it was not wrong for a married man to sleep with an unmarried woman, because he then was expected to marry her, and polygamy was permissible.[65] Of course, as in every other society, promiscuity existed; young men would have different girl-friends before marriage. The existence of the phenomenon was commonly known but quietly tolerated. Whereas it was acknowledged that young men had to acquire experience before they got married, young girls were expected to be virgins until their wedding-night. Sempebwa modifies this rule however. According to him, premarital sex, since it does not involve the basic value of fertility, has no moral connotations. If the bride is found not to be a virgin, this is no reason for divorce.[66] The Kabaka's pamphlet undermines that view: "It was one of the worst filial offence for a daughter to become pregnant while living with her parents. As soon as she was discovered in that condition she was at once expelled from her parents' house,... This custom was intended to stimulate morality among the Baganda girls, since any girl who went astray before she was given in marriage suffered this indignity and was always looked upon with contempt by all her relatives and friends."[67] Only when the girl was found to be pregnant, she was expelled. The concept of virginity is not mentioned by the Kabaka.

According to Ganda customary law, affairs outside marriage were not acceptable. Polygamy however was and remains accepted which conflicts with the Christian demand for monogamy. To the missionaries, traditional Ganda society appeared promiscuous whereas to the Baganda themselves, life was defined according to a rigid and functioning moral system. These different notions are evident in the explanations Winifred Brown, wife of

---

63 s.a. Joshua W. Sempebwa, *African Traditional Moral Norms and Their Implication for Christianity. A Case Study of Ganda Ethics* (St. Augustin: Steyler Verlag, 1983), p. 90-1.

64 The seriousness that was attached to adultery as offence becomes clear when keeping in mind that in the 19th century, the punishment for adultery was death; s.a. Walter Rusch, *Klassen und Staat in Buganda vor der Kolonialzeit, Veröffentlichungen des Museums für Völkerkunde zu Leipzig. Heft 25* (Berlin: Akademie Verlag, 1975), p. 292.

65 Sempebwa, *African Traditional Moral Norms*, p. 91.

66 ibid., p. 91.

67 The Kabaka's pamphlet, p. 106.

the Anglican Bishop and later Archbishop put forward as late as 1988 to account for the rise of promiscuity and prostitution. She points out that in a society with approximately equal numbers of men and women, as is the case in Uganda, the balance is upset when some men take more than one wife. Not enough women are left for every man to have one, which means that several men have to share one woman, and thus "polygamy gives rise to promiscuity, and to prostitution as a lucrative profession..."[68] As another reason for the rise of promiscuity, Brown cites the war with its decline of moral values. Her argumentation shows that even people who understand the different social concepts develop seemingly logic arguments in order to justify the Christian viewpoint that equates promisquity with polygamy. It is important to keep in mind that the Ugandan concept promiscuity refers to prostitution, not to polygamy. It makes sense, therefore, to represent promiscuity as something bad, and to suggest going back to the original system of norms and values. Polygamy would remain a safe sexual behaviour, as long as everybody observed the rules and had no sexual relationships outside the marriage.

Owing to interactions between the cultures, and also to the influence of Christianity, these two notions are confused by both Westerners and Ugandans. Nevertheless, it appears important to state them, because they have a direct impact on the effectiveness of a play.[69]

3.6.2. Urbanisation

Traditional Ganda society as it existed before colonialism, has disintegrated. Twenty years of civil war and migration to towns have had its effects on the structure of society. During the war, thousands of people were killed and many others had to leave their areas because life had become unsafe. Social structures in the rural areas were disrupted, and the means of production in those areas, like fields and coffee-plantations were destroyed.[70] Most survivors found themselves in a difficult economic situation after the war. Many young men migrated into urban areas, primarily to Kampala. In Uganda, industry is situated in the urban centres in the south where the

68 Winifred Brown, *Marriage, Divorce and Inheritance. The Uganda Council of Women's Movement for Legislative Reform* (Cambridge African Monographs 10. Cambridge: African Studies Centre, 1988), p. 3. The Browns lived in Kampala between 1953 and 1965.

69 for a more detailed discussion of the overlapping of those notions, s. chapter 3.6.1.

70 What has happened in the Luweero District exemplifies the situation; s. p. 64.

infrastructure is better developed. Consequently, the urban centres have become the focal point of migrants from the rural areas who are looking for jobs. As far as work is concerned, industrialisation has contributed to an even more pronounced polarisation between urban and rural centres.[71]

Although it is mainly for economic reasons that people leave the rural areas, there are also other, noneconomic factors that contribute to this migration. Polls carried out by Richard Marvin have revealed the poor rural infrastructure is one of them.[72] Electricity and transport systems in the villages are bad, and health facilities are not sufficient. David W. Dunlop points out that in 1973 the proportion of health services employment was approximately fifty-nine per cent larger in the towns than in the districts.[73] Although this figure dates back 20 years, the problem of health facilities in the rural areas of Uganda is still prevalent today. Other factors mentioned in the poll were better trading facilities in the towns, commerce, food, security, accessibility to news and knowledge, and entertainment.

It is hardly surprising that, especially in the cities, there is a high incidence of prostitution. Many men who come to work there leave their families in the villages and turn to prostitutes for sexual gratification. Many women are forced into prostitution for survival when their marriages in the city, deprived of the social support system of the village, fail. Prostitution is one of the few options they have to survive economically. Accordingly, in Marvin's poll, prostitution was seen as a danger to both men and women in the cities. Several times, the need for money was cited as a cause for it:

> If somebody is sent from his father's home he or she goes and lives in the town. But when she is a girl what she does is to go and hire a house and when she sees that she hasn't enough money she starts selling herself. I mean to be a bar maid. If somebody continues with that habit that means that our country is losing youngsters.[74]

---

71 Axel J. Halbach, *Industriestruktur und Industrialisierungspolitik in Uganda, 1963-1972*, IFO-Institut für Wirtschaftsforschung (München. Forschungsberichte der Afrikastudienstelle 50. München: Weltforum Verlag, 1974), p. 184.

72 Richard Marvin, *Land of Wages. The Evaluation of Occupational and Residential Alternatives by the Rural Basoga*, IFO-Institut für Wirtschaftsforschung (München. Afrika-Studien 101. München, London: Weltforum Verlag, 1978), p. 79 ff.

73 David W. Dunlop, *The Economic of Uganda's Health Service System: Implications for Health and Economic Planning*, Diss. Michigan State University 1973, (Ann Arbor, Michigan: University Microfilms International, 1973), p. 238.

74 quoted in Marvin, *Land of Wages*, p. 87.

Other women come from the villages, because they want to break with traditional values. In Ganda society, the female sex is regarded to be weaker than the male one, needing both the man's protection and authority.[75] Women are subordinated. First, to their parents, who may also choose the husband for the daughter; second, they have to obey the husbands.

Not surprisingly, in melting pots like Kampala, both men and women have sex with multiple partners. It is important to reiterate that Ugandans regard this practice as immoral, while the traditional polygamous household was considered morally correct.

3.6.3. Social Structure

Traditionally, Ganda society was structured according to a strict hierarchy with God at the top. After Him came the spirits of the dead, and then, in the realm of the living, the *Kabaka* (King). Sempebwa explains the Baganda conceive things in a hierarchical relation to other things.[76] Power is viewed hierarchically and age is coupled with rank since old people are closer to the world of the spirits. Age, therefore, conveys authority. When two or more Baganda are involved in any kind of social relationship, their position in the hierarchy is of utmost relevance to the relationship - and, as Sempebwa points out, in almost any human relation among the Baganda there is some sort of superiority of one actor over the other. Subordination therefore is essential, but without subservience. Nobody is merely instrumental to serve the well-being of the one higher in the hierarchy. Each benefits from the other, and each has a vital role to play in the life of the other.[77] The principle of human hierarchy constitutes one of the three basic principles in traditional Ganda society, from which all other moral rules derive.[78] Even after Obote had abolished the Kingdoms in 1967, that hierarchical structure remained intact. Concepts as 'talking back' did and do not exist. This is also reflected in the education of the children who from early childhood on are taught the rules of obedience towards elders and superiors. Musujju thus writes: "Obedience is a virtue greatly cherished among the Ganda... right when the child started to speak the parents taught him/her to be obedient

---

75 Sempebwa, *Traditional African Moral Norms*, p. 162.

76 ibid., p. 60.

77 ibid., p. 66 ff.

78 The two other basic principles in Ganda traditional society are those of human solidarity and oneness; human vitality and continuity.

to the elders and the child grew up in an atmosphere of obedience because he/she saw the mother obedient to the father, the father to the village chief, the village chief to the *muluka* (sub-district) chief, the *muluka* chief to the *gombolola* (sub-county) chief, the *gombolola* to the *saza* (county) chief, the *saza* chief to the *Kabaka*."[79] The prescription of respect to those older in age is applied in all interpersonal relationships. Parents and other relatives impart knowledge they consider relevant to the children, and it is expected that the children absorb that knowledge without comments; questions are not encouraged.[80] Similarly, adults display this behaviour with their superiors either at work or in the family. Knowledge and information is thereby handed down from the top of the hierarchy.

When looking at the communication between NGOs, international organisations, playwrights, actors and audience, it becomes clear that the situation is asymetric. This is however not only the case between NGOs and international organisations on the one side and artists on the other. One has to consider the possibility that the social attitude towards hierarchical relationships is also the basic notion of those Ugandan artists who produce TFD plays. Of course, that concept also serves the purpose of international organisations and NGOs who want to convince the audience of their ideas about how to prevent the further spreading of AIDS. They apply it themselves in their workshops when they brief the artists on the kind of information to be passed on to the audiences. It seems, however, too superficial to talk of asymmetric communication on the side of the international organisations and NGOs only. While it is undoubtedly true that they encourage discussions only in the workshops, and only for the purpose of appearing to communicate in a symmetrical way, it also has to be born in mind that there is a similar attitude on the Ugandan side. It would be interesting to investigate if the Ugandan artists who attend the workshops and who create the plays afterwards have, although subconsciously, the notion of 'talking-down' as an effective way of communicating in their society. Apparently, CT follows that tradition of spreading information.

A strict hierarchical structure of a society leads to the development of certain patterns of behaviour - a mechanism which may be assumed as given

[79] quoted in Sempebwa, *Traditional African Moral Norms*, p. 118.

[80] Conversation with K. Matovu, lecturer in the Department of Luganda, Makerere University, Kampala/Uganda, September 1991.

for Ganda society. In a society where it is expected to receive information and orders passively, people have to find means to still do what they want without appearing to be opposing the instructions given to them. After all, we are dealing with adults who have their own thoughts which may not coincide with orders coming from the top of society. It is likely that the rules of obedience existing in Ganda society create an attitude in the population of accepting orders and information without many questions, but still doing what they want to do. It is difficult to say anything definite about an area as sensitive as AIDS where the sexual habits of a society are involved. Sexual behaviour as form of social behaviour is probably functioning according to stricter rules than any other area of social intercourse. Moreover, behaviour that is motivated by sexual urge, does not follow rational thought patterns. Maybe, this helps explain the AIDS-problem. As a result of the many AIDS information campaigns in the country, there is already a high level of awareness about the disease among Ugandans. Nevertheless, AIDS is spreading - which may have to do with social factors as well as with the fact that the population does not draw the necessary conclusion from the information campaigns to change their own sexual behaviour. It almost seems as if the information given in plays is regarded like other orders coming from the top, where one has the possibility of not acting accordingly. Another explanation which is even more likely might be that most people believe to adhere to conformity under moral rules, but are still leading a "promiscuous" life despite the warning, due to the fact that they regard their own situation as the exception. They are either convinced that their partners are not infected with AIDS; or they simply do not regard their behaviour as promiscuous. In all probability, both mechanisms - patterns of evasions and claims for the own exceptional situation - are at work here. This may account for why people have not changed their behaviour although they are given the information and incentive to do so.

3.6.4. Attitude Towards Age

Another point to consider is the concept of age in Ganda society. In Europe and the United States, it is reasonable to expect to live to the age of 70 if not longer. In Uganda, however, life expectancy is much lower. Until colonialism, medical treatment, as elsewhere in the "Third World," was not so efficient and well developed. People died young of diseases like malaria, diarrhoea etc., and there was a high infant mortality rate. The situation improved slightly with colonialism. Trained medical personnel and drugs came into the country, which was mainly done for the benefit of the British soldiers. The Ugandan population, however, also profited by it. Still, life expectancy was considerably lower than in Europe, and it did not rise after independence either - rather on the contrary. During the 20 years of Civil war the infrastructure in the country was destroyed, and medical treatment was almost non-existent. Besides, thousands of people in the villages and rural areas were killed by both army and secret police under Obote and Amin. What happened in Luweero typifies the situation during that time.[81]

As a result of twenty years of Civil war, there is in Uganda today a generation which grew up with the notion that it is normal to die at age 30 or 40. There is no awareness that one can live longer by protecting one's health, so for people it does not really matter in the end if they die of AIDS or any other disease. Besides, the idea of death in Ganda culture is not as frightening as it is in the West. Death does not mean the end of life, but rather its continuation in the world of the spirits who have a higher position in the social hierarchy.[82]

It appears this problem is not reflected in the plays about AIDS. The producers of the plays erroneously assume that everybody expects to become old and is willing to take care of one's health. That audiences are more fatalistic with regard to their life expectancy is ignored, and this attitude is among the first things that will have to be changed when trying to raise the people's awareness about AIDS. Initially, the audience has to be convinced it is indeed possible and desirable to grow old. Without this attitude, it is useless to give information about the prevention of AIDS or condom use. The information will not lead to behavioural change, so long as the audience does not have the basic consciousness about the desirability of old age. Paulo Freire also stresses the need for the creation of an awareness of reality as a historical moment which is subject to change. He explains that all people live in a dialectic relationship between the determination of limits and their own freedom: "As they seperate themselves from the world, which they objectify, as they seperate themselves from their own activity, as they locate the seat of their decisions in themselves and in their relations with the world and others, men overcome the situations which limit them: the 'limit-situations.'"[83] Once men perceive of those limit-situations as obstacles

81 s.p. 64.

82 Sempebwa, *Traditional African Moral Norms*, p.48 and 57 ff.

83 Freire, *Pedagogy of the Oppressed*, p. 71.

to their liberation, they react to them with 'limit-acts,'[84] thus revealing that the limits are historical dimensions of a given reality. It is not the limit-situations themselves that create a climate of hopelessness, but rather how they are perceived by men at a historical moment: "whether they appear as fetters or insurmountable barriers."[85] Only when a climate of hope and an awareness of the possibility for change is created, men try to overcome the limit-situations.

After having presented those social concepts of Ganda society that are relevant to an understanding of Campaign Theatre against AIDS, I will continue the discussion of the phenomenon CT itself. In a first chapter on the communicator I will describe the typical organisational structures as they have emerged in CT over the last three to four years.

3.7. The Communicator

That the focus in the fight against AIDS is on large, spectacular information-campaigns results from the fact that international organisations and NGOs, with their own internal pressures, are involved. After 20 years of almost complete isolation, and with many current problems Uganda is a welcome new field for development organisations. Since the war ended in 1986, more and more of them have channelled money into the country - a big part of it for the fight against AIDS.[86] The money has to be spent, and there must be, if possible, immediate and quantifiable results to account for its use. Big information campaigns in that respect serve the purpose of reaching many people so that the educative message is spread most widely, and they bring measurable data in form of numbers of spectators. Relying on audience figures as measure for success may, however, lead to self-delusion. Spectacular events like the AIDS Quake Festival are well-attended and therefore appear successful for the organisers in their reports to headquarters, which gives more money to be spent in more information campaigns.[87]

---

84 Vieira Pinta, quoted in Freire, *Pedagogy of the Oppressed*, p. 72.

85 Freire, *Pedagogy of the Oppressed*, p. 72.

86 The majority of external funding still goes into agriculture and infrastructural development.

87 Obviously, this only holds true for the PR-side of the fight against AIDS; organisations like WHO, UNICEF etc. spend a lot of their money for research and treatment, and for workshops who train local health educators.

With CT, one cannot speak of a single communicator. What we have is rather a chain of communicators. At the beginning of the chain quite often is an international organisation or an NGO with external funding. According to the principle 'train the trainers,' they organise workshops for Ugandan artists and performers where they brief them on facts about AIDS: methods of transmission, prevention/protection, treatment of those who are already infected etc. With knowledge thus acquired in the workshops, the artists then create plays which are performed by actors. Each element in the chain has a different function. The international organisation contributes both facts and money. With the information they dispense they try, through the playwrights and actors, to influence the Ugandan population to change their behaviour. Generally speaking, influence will lead to a change or reversal of previous (or predicted) decisions, policies, or behaviour.[88] In order to influence people, some sort of power has to be exercised. Many sociologists and political scientists accordingly see a clear connection between influence and power. Merton thinks that the two concepts are closely related but not identical, since "power, prestige, position in a hierarchy etc. may contribute to the potential for interpersonal influence, but do not determine the extend to which influence actually occurs."[89] For B. Russell, on the other hand, who defines power as the production of intended effects, they are identical. C.J. Friedrich's definition of influence as a 'very evasive' form of power has found wide acceptance. This definition is also suitable to describe the communication between NGOs or international organisations, and the artists and the audience. Obviously, an asymmetrical relationship is involved wherever influence is exercised. The influence exercised by international organisations is a very evasive form of power, since the "change of behaviour of the influenced is due to advice, manipulation, imitation, and the like, instead of coercion or the exercise of formal authority."[90] The Ugandan artists are supposed to use both money and information donated from the NGOs and organisations to create plays.[91] In addition to that, however, they bring in the Ugandan component so that the plays succeed in appealing to cognitive and affective systems of

---

88 Julius Gould and William L. Kolb, ed, *A Dictionary of the Social Sciences. Compiled under the auspices of the United Nations Educational, Scientific, and Cultural Organisation* (New York: the Free Press, 1988).

89 ibid., p. 332.

90 ibid., p. 333.

91 The choice as to what kind of plays they create is left to them; once the workshops are over the organisations, to my knowledge, do not influence the work of the artists.

the audience.[92] This can only be done by members of the same culture, not by outsiders. The artists use the material in form of informations from the workshops and relate it to the Ugandan context, e.g., they use forms, techniques and language relevant to a Ugandan audience. The actors, finally, have to present the play in such a way that the audience catches the message. They have to be entertaining without letting the message be blurred by the entertainment aspect of the show. They are the mediators between the audience and the information to be disseminated.

The communication situation as it occurs in CT is asymmetric since the information is passed down from the top. International organisations have the money and the organisational framework to both acquire factual information through research as well as to pass the information on to the next element in the chain. In the workshops, however, the communication is made to appear symmetric. The artists are encouraged to ask questions and discuss the information conveyed to them by the workshop organisers. An asymmetric situation is thereby transferred into a symmetric one by giving the impression of arriving at conclusions in a joint effort. This device, applied in workshops, seminars, and didactic situations, serves various purposes: the participants feel involved and do not have the impression of being patronized. By actively participating they internalise the information better than through a lecture. Besides, the artists are thus trained for discussions with the audiences after the performances. The questions and comments coming from the participants in the workshop, may very well be those coming from the spectators after the play. At the end of the workshop, the artists are supposed to feel confident about their level of information and their ability to communicate to their audience effectively. The workshops, besides passing along information, also represent a means to train the actors for discussions and instill a feeling of superiority in them. The direct influence of the international organisation stops, once the workshop is over. It is then up to the artists and playwrights to find the right way of conveying their message. The organisers of the workshop must therefore try to convince the artists of their viewpoint while the seminar lasts.

With this kind of asymmetric communication, the basic principle is that of a difference in *niveau*. The international organisations and NGOs perceive the artists as uninformed, and the playwrights in turn have that

---

92 for a detailed discussion, s. chapter 3.8.

conception of their audience. Besides the general assumption of different levels of awareness, there is also the difference between rural areas and the towns. The population in rural areas is stereotypically associated with inflexible reduced attitudes, whereas the inhabitants in towns are expected to be more open-minded and flexible, which may be one of the reasons CT concentrates on the towns. In addition, there are other more pragmatic reasons. The international organisations usually hold their workshops in Kampala, where they have their offices, or in one of the major towns in the south of Uganda. The artists who attend the workshops, therefore are from Kampala, Jinja, Masaka, Entebbe, etc., and perform in those areas. Due to this focus on the more accessible areas in the south, the situation arises that more and more information reaches people in those districts, whereas the population in rural areas is comparatively neglected.

A final point concerns the international organisations and the question what they realistically can achieve. It seems to me mistaken to accuse them of not taking the social causes to which the problem AIDS is connected into account. People who introduce that argument usually draw attention to the fact that the spreading of AIDS has to do with poverty. The population of a poor country like Uganda does not have the opportunity to pick up information and to protect itself as people from rich countries do. Another point is that the general medical status in poor countries is much lower than in industrialized countries.[93] Medical treatment is expensive, and unless absolutely necessary, Ugandans tend not to see a doctor because they do not have the money to pay for the treatment. Even then, vital drugs and equipment are not available. Consequently they do not get treatment for diseases like genital ulcer and other STDs which enhances the chance of infection with AIDS through sexual intercourse. The progression from HIV to AIDS for an HIV-positive European takes much longer than for a Ugandan - simply because his/her general physical condition is stronger, owing to diet and general care for his/her well-being. However desirable it may be, it is not realistic to demand the elimination of the social causes of the disease all at once. This is a slow process which can only progress in small steps. One of the steps is the effort of international organisations and NGOs to try to create a consciousness in Ugandans for health care and to give them necessary information about AIDS protection. As the discussion in the next chapter will show, this is not always successful. One reason for

93 In Uganda, for example, the average annual medical expenditure per capita is less than 50 cents.

the failure is the ignorance of social and cultural concepts of Ganda society. Another reason, in my opinion, is the appeal of religious NGOs and the Churches to Western moral norms like monogamy. If Ugandans are to be convinced to reduce the risk of HIV-infection by a reduction of sexual contacts to one partner, it has to be done by developing arguments from within the Ganda moral system, and not by arguing according to Western/Christian moral norms.

As will be seen in more detail in the discussion of the case studies, theatre plays that try to raise consciousness for the fight against AIDS apply certain techniques that appeal to the audience's consciousness. In order to understand how those techniques work, in the following chapter a closer look at such sociological concepts as consciousness, learning, internalisation, change of behaviour, will be taken. Those concepts will be discussed in the context of the Ugandan situation.

3.8. The Raising of Consciousness

The consciousness of individuals is based on the value system of society. Ellingsworth and Rokeach both point out that beliefs have a cultural base growing out of nurture and conditioning. Similarities of belief, therefore, are shared by members of a community.[94] The individual's consciousness and behaviour are thus shaped by the culture in which it lives. There exists a multitude of definitions of culture from various disciplines. For this study, a fairly general definition seems most useful: culture consists of "patterns, explicit and implicit, of and for behaviour acquired and transmitted by symbols, constituting the distinctive achievements of human groups, including their embodiments in artifacts; the essential core of culture consists of traditional (i.e. historically derived and selected) ideas and especially their attached values; culture systems may, on the one hand, be considered as products of action, on the other as conditioning elements of further action."[95] The consciousness of individuals, shaped by their respective culture, is composed of various elements, like the awareness of one's own mental and bodily functions, the awareness of objects in the external world, the perception of oneself as an individuality, and the

94 Milton Rokeach, *The Nature of Human Values* (New York: Free Press, 1973), pp. 121-25; Huber Ellingsworth, "Adaptive Intercultural Communication," p. 197.

95 "Culture: A Critical Review of Concepts and Definitions," Papers of the Peabody Museum of American Archeology and Ethnology, vol. 47, no. 1, 1952, p. 181; in *A Dictionary of the Social Sciences*, p. 165.

perception of oneself as a member of a group. Consciousness does not exist without its opposition, unconsciousness. Many sociologists in fact define consciousness by its comparison to the unconscious.[96] Consciousness would then be the continuous, clearly shaped rational part of mental life, where mental energy is transformed by verbal symbols. Unconscious experiences, on the other hand, are discontinuous, vague, inarticulate and irrational.[97] Rokeach describes the human consciousness as a belief system consisting of three parts: *cognitive beliefs* represent a person's knowledge and the degree of agreement or disagreement with that knowledge; *affective beliefs* underlie degree of arousal about an object as concept; and *behavioural beliefs* predispose to action. The three beliefs are inseparable and interactive, and together they constitute the "total cognitive universe of a person's beliefs about the social world and his or her self."[98]

When trying to change the consciousness of people, one must bear in mind that human behaviour is viewed to be influenced by basically two aspects of culture. One aspect is 'objective culture' containing such factors as names (concepts) of things, ethnicity, gender, age, education, economic background, employment, and housing. Those factors are recognizable characteristics of people in a certain social environment. The other aspect is 'subjective culture' which contains social factors such as feeling, believing, conceiving, judging, hoping, intending, and meaning. These factors represent mental characteristics and cannot be immediately observed. The two aspects are interactive and involve evaluation processes and behavioural intentions with respect to various life experiences. Tzeng et al. explain that individuals assimilate the subjective characteristics of each culture and consequently develop two systems: the cognitive system which represents a person's descriptive attributions of objects and events, and the affective

96 In the *Theses*, Uspenskij et al. define culture as inseperably linked with its opposition, "non-culture." Culture would then be the sphere of organisation in human society and its oppostion, disorganisation. The authors state that a characteristic of the twentieth century is that the reserves of the spatial expansion of culture have been exhausted (all geographical space has become "cultural"). That is why scholars in our century have addressed themselves to the problem of the subconscious, thus constructing a new type of space opposed to culture. Uspenskij et al. consider the opposition between the spheres of the subconscious and those of the cosmos as essential to an understanding of the inner structure of twentieth-century culture. For a more detailed discussion, s. Uspenskij et al., "Theses on the Semiotic Study of Culture"; Winner, "the Semiotics of Cultural Texts"; Winner "Ethnicity, Modernity, and Theory of Culture Texts."

97 *A Dictionary of the Social Sciences*, p. 127.

98 Ellingsworth, "Adaptive Intercultural Communication," p. 197.

system, representing a person's emotional and autonomous attributions towards objects.[99] They draw attention to the fact that affective attribution usually includes semantic generalisations across a wide range of life contexts and situations, and therefore influences the individual's overt behaviours and dispositions to a large extent. When trying to raise consciousness in order to change behaviour, therefore, both systems, the cognitive as well as the affective have to be addressed. Evidently, this cannot be done by applying the same methods.[100]

Changes of behaviour are the result of learning, which is "the process by which an activity originates or is changed through reacting to an encountered situation, provided that the characteristics of the change in activity cannot be explained on the basis of native response tendencies, maturation, or temporary stages of the organism (e.g. fatigue, drugs, etc.)."[101] Another form of learning is internalisation which, according to psycho-analytic definition, occurs when the learner is unaware of the conditions which motivated his learning. Internalisation is involved when the super-ego's contents are acquired, like e.g. moral norms and conscience.[102] In the case of TFD plays which inform about the prevention of AIDS, the ultimate aim is for the audience to internalise the message suggesting a change of behaviour. When trying to organise an information campaign therefore, the first question the communicators have to ask themselves is the relationship between the consciousness prevalent in society, constituted by the factors mentioned, and the 'new' consciousness they want the audience to adopt.

An information campaign starts when a situation occurs that has to be solved by a change of behaviour. In Uganda, this was the case when the rising number of AIDS infections was realised. The disease affects everybody, including children whose parents have died of AIDS or who were themselves infected in the womb. All Ugandans have lost friends or relatives to AIDS. Whereas the Ugandan population has responded rather fatalistically to this new threat to their lives, GOs, NGOs and international

---

99 O. Tzeng, C.J. Duvall, Roger Ware, Robert Neel and Robert Fortier, "Subjective Intergroup Distances of Blacks and Whites," in *Interethnic Communication. Current Research*, ed. Zoung Yun Kim (Newbury Park, Beverly Hills, London, New Delhi: Sage Publications, 1986), p. 61 ff.

100 for a detailed discussion, s. chapter 3.8.1.

101 *Theories of Learning* (New York: Appleton, Century-Crofts, 2nd edn., 1956, p. 3) in *A Dictionary of the Social Sciences*, p. 381.

102 ibid., p. 345.

organisations realise the further spreading of the disease must be stopped. By 1988/89, the number of infections had grown so fast that it aroused world-wide concern and caused international organisations like UNICEF, WHO, Red Cross etc. to come to Uganda, and contribute large sums of money to the fight against AIDS. It seems that the efforts of those involved in this work have taken two directions: to prevent the further spreading of the disease, and to find ways of living with those Ugandans who are already infected - a large number by now. In both instances, it was necessary to create an awareness of the problem in the population. This was and is done through information campaigns using media like radio, TV, newspapers, posters, tapes, videos and theatre. Theatre especially, with its direct exchange between actors and audience, plays a crucial role here.[103] GOs, NGOs and international organisations understand theatre is an ideal medium to spread information in a country with little media-infrastructure, and to reinforce the message in discussions with the audience.

Emphasis is placed on the presentation of the disease as a social rather than an individual threat. The plays pass the message that Ugandans have the social responsibility to protect the children by not spreading AIDS further. It is made explicitly clear that AIDS is transmitted mainly by sexual intercourse, and that multiple partners lead to a high risk of infection and transmission. That means both groups, those who are not yet infected as well as those who are already HIV-positive, have to live responsibly, i.e. have one sexual partner and use condoms.

The plays express the view that promiscuity is morally bad - even more so because it is the main cause for AIDS. They also stress, however, that those people who are already infected must not be stigmatised. The appeal to morality is made in order to influence the behaviour of society from now on. There is no moral judgement on those who are already infected. In fact, the plays explicitly admonish the audience not to regard AIDS-patients as morally bad. It is made clear that they can still lead a useful life and have to remain integrated into society. Obviously, when applying the concept of morality as an argument against promiscuity a particular effort has to be made to keep the two arguments separated: promiscuity which is regarded as morally bad, and the necessity not to stigmatise AIDS-patients.

---

[103] s. chapter 3.5.

The goal of TFD, i.e. the changing of behaviour is classified by Doob as a social goal, because the emphasis is on affecting other people.[104] Social goals are involved in all kinds of training, like child-rearing and general education concerning the rules and values of society etc. With a social goal as basis, the dominant motive to communicate in TFD is to convey information about AIDS rather than to entertain the audience; entertainment arising out of the play is an incidental goal. It is used as an instrument to catch the interest of the spectators and as such enhance the chance of having them internalise the message.

The plays work on the affective and the cognitive systems of the audience. On the affective level, they try to shock the spectators out of complacency. On the cognitive level, the communicators want to provoke rational thought processes in the audience that would eventually cause a lasting change of behaviour.[105] Doob draws attention to the fact, however, that there frequently are unintended goals which may be even more important than the intended ones. The communicator may be unaware of some of the consequences of his communication. A play on AIDS which is intended to educate the audience, could be mistaken for entertainment by the spetators who do not perceive the information as the dominating goal; or concepts may be mentioned in the play that are foreign to the culture and therefore will be misunderstood. As an example, Mkanju states that a group that wants to perform to a Maasai community and has "infection by syringes" in its programme, may be counter productive.[106] The needle drug culture is not a problem in the area, and the only persons who have needles are doctors and nurses. When the actors talk about infection through needles, the people in the area may just not go to the hospital anymore for fear to be infected with AIDS through injections. The message of a TFD-play has to be relevant, otherwise there may be results contrary to the ones hoped for.

Especially with plays that are produced by outsiders, the risk of such misunderstandings is high. In Uganda, in order to diminish the risk, the plays are usually developed by Ugandan artists creating a situation where TFD plays as a thought-construct, are endogenous. There are, however,

---

104 Social goals are opposed to the so called primary goals which involve the bare survival of people, s. Doob, *Communication in Africa*, p. 40.

105 Intended goal is the goal which motivates the communicator and which he can report to himself and to others; ibid., p. 49.

106 Mkanju, in *The Sunday Nation* (Kenya), August 25th, 1991.

exogenous factors when the project is transformed into reality, e.g. funding from international organisations, briefing in workshops, venues etc. In the plays, therefore, the problem is not entirely defined by the target group itself. Although they are created and performed by Ugandan artists, the information that is supposed to be given comes from outsiders, e.g. medical doctors, often belonging to one of the international organisations or NGOs. The members of those organisations in turn, are responsible to their headquarters in Europe and the U.S. The definition of the problem, as well as the perception as to what is the wrong and what the right kind of behaviour is therefore influenced to a large extent from outside. Unlike with project-oriented plays, where one project is implemented by the target group with the help of TFD, and with comparatively little money, in information campaigns, the dimensions are much bigger.[107]

All plays about AIDS try to instill an awareness that it is not too late for change. Although many people already suffer from the disease, there is still a chance to save others, especially the children and uninfected adults. The plays are based on the assumption that the audience knows about the disease but has not yet done anything to prevent its further spreading; it is necessary to educate them and create an awareness of their individual ability to act and take responsibility. The awareness of AIDS as a problem is high, but combined with a fatalistic attitude towards it, and international organisations and NGOs came to modify that attitude.

Like the project-oriented plays already discussed, the plays must aim at making the spectators recognise the threat to their individual lives, as well as their social responsibility to change their behaviour for the benefit of the nation. This is based on the notion that, according to the Ganda principle of human vitality and continuity, man as a unique individual is less important than man as a link in the chain of generations. Each individual is "part of the great stream of the continuous vitalistic life that transcends his own self."[108] This view obligates everyone to promote the well-being of others, and to participate vitally in the continual flow of life. The only actions which are morally worthy are those directed towards realizing the ideals of human vitality and continuity.[109] The individual cannot exist alone. He/she owes his/her existence to others and is part of a whole. People are consequently

[107] for a detailed discussion, s. chapters 3.7. and 3.8.1.

[108] Sempebwa, *Traditional African Moral Norms*, p. 59.

[109] ibid., p. 59.

expected to care not only for their own family and clan, but also for neighbours. Human solidarity is regarded as one of the highest ideals. Since there is little room for individual decisions, a change of behaviour can only be achieved by appeals to the responsibility for the other members of society. When AIDS is presented as a social problem rather than an individual or purely medical one, it makes society at large responsible for solving it. It may be assumed as given the producers of the plays against AIDS - in most cases Ugandans - either have this element of Ganda world-view consciously in mind, or, subconsciously, have interanlized it as members of Ganda society.

3.8.1. The Communication

When regarding communication in form of plays, there are certain questions that have to be born in mind: What is the content of the communication? What does it say or attempt to say? How is the message expressed? What is its style? Which techniques are applied? In what language is the play performed? What are some of the attributes of that language? In this discussion of the communication, the focus will concentrate on such theoretical concepts as the content of the plays in relation to their effect in the consciousness of the audience. The more practical phenomena, such as the forms and techniques applied by the producers of the plays and which are based on *their* conception of the audience's consciousness, will be discussed in detail in the case studies.

First, there is purely medical information about channels of infection and prevention; these are verifiable facts and not to be disputed. With information, the plays clearly aim at the cognitive consciousness of the audience. On a rational basis, scientific information is conveyed to the spectators giving them the knowledge to behave correctly and responsibly.

Secondly, the plays work on an emotional level, thereby appealing to the affective system. The audience is shocked by what it sees. In the plays, there is always a representation of a bad example, e.g. multiple sexual partners or spreading the disease to uninfected people. In one of the plays, *It's Not Easy*, a husband infects his wife, and she in turn passes the disease on to their baby. The problem of AIDS in this play is exemplified through the individual fate of one family. When watching the play, the spectators duplicate the action emotionally and realise what is happening on stage could easily happen to them too. They are shocked in two respects: through emotional identification with the fate of the fictional characters on stage, and by the realization that the same could happen to them.

On the emotional level too, the plays pass the message that AIDS has spread so quickly because of a promiscuous life style. All the plays stress the immorality of promiscuity, and that it is the reason for the spread of AIDS. The moral judgement that promiscuity is bad is therefore brought into connection with the health risk. As a solution to the problem, the plays suggest a return to "correct" moral behaviour: stop having sex with different partners, lead a monogamous life. The plays implicitly refer to the traditional moral system that has been abandoned, due to the social and political problems the country has had over the last 20 years. The ultimate message of the information campaigns, therefore, is not really to change the consciousness of the population - rather to create an awareness they have diverted from the right moral behaviour, and they now must go back to it. This rhetoric implies that what is necessary to solve the problem of AIDS is not as difficult as it seems. Society once was on the right way - all that is needed now, is to go back to it.

The fact that the cognitive and the affective system are interactive is taken into account in the plays, as the appeals to both systems are intertwined. The risk of getting infected with AIDS is coupled with the moral judgement on promiscuity. At the same time they are made to draw the rational conclusion that if they as individuals behave irresponsibly, then society as a whole is affected. The plays therefore attempt to initiate the interdependent mechanisms of both cognitive and affective system.

Although other causes of AIDS, such as infection through blood-transfusions, needles, tatooing, circumcision etc., are discussed in the workshops preceding the plays, they are not mentioned in the plays, for a number of reasons. One is that a situation has to be presented on stage in which individual behaviour is decisive and thereby enables spectators to draw parallels with their own behaviour. A love-story serves that purpose better than a story in which somebody gets infected through a blood-transfusion. A love-story refers to experiences most people have, whereas with any other topic, the majority of the spectators may not feel that those situations play a part in their lives. The stress on promiscuity takes into account the necessity the plays must represent situations familiar to the spectators so they can recognise them as being relevant. Love-stories have the advantage of being neither too explicit nor too enigmatic - everybody in the audience can identify with the plot.[110] With the stress on promiscuity it is possible to involve the affective system of the spectators to a larger extent, because their own sense of morality is addressed. Wrong moral behaviour is depicted so the audience can reach the conclusion that it is necessary to return to the right moral values. The device of over-emphasising the negative is based on the realization that negative behaviour is more informative and carries greater weight by standing in contrast to standards of behaviour and expectations emphasizing the positive. In the attribution process, deviations from the norm are more revealing than conformity with it.[111] The main reason for the apparent focus on promiscuity is the fact, that it actually is the major channel for spreading the disease, and as such has to be repeatedly stressed.

An important aspect of a communication through TFD is entertainment. The primary goal of a didactic play is to spread the message that will create a new awareness in the audience. In order to both arouse and keep the interest of the spectators, however, the play has to be entertaining as well. Very often in the Ugandan TFD plays, entertainment derives from humour. Producers take care, however, that there is just enough humour to entertain the audience, not more:

> Humour: should be kept to a minimum to create just enough entertainment. Too much of it during a performance can turn a (didactic) developmental play into a farce. It was noted that too much humour can create long noisy periods by the audience which distorts the overall presentation. This goes for 'very rich' instrumental accompaniments in songs which may draw the audience's attention more than the message in the song.[112]

There are plays which have AIDS as their dominant topic, whereas in other plays reference to the disease is just made in one short episode. Only those plays created to inform and educate, and therefore have AIDS as their dominant topic, will be categorised as TFD where every element of the play, structure, music, songs etc. serves the educational purpose.

There are some inherent contradictions in the plays about AIDS. Even though they all appeal to the traditional system of Ganda moral norms, they confuse some of the traditional concepts with those of the West.

---

110 This follows Freire's demand that the codifications must represent situations familiar to the individuals whose thematics are being examined. S. *Pedagogy of the Oppressed*, p. 76.

111 Kanouse and Hanson, in Ehrenhaus, "Culture and the Attribution Process," p. 267.

112 Muganga, "The Nattyole Experience," p. 13.

Promiscuity in the Western sense is confused with the Ugandan notion of promiscuity, which clearly allows for polygamy. If a play advocates monogamy by appealing to traditional (polygamous) Ganda culture, it is unlikely to create much of an effect, whereas the argument in favour of faithfulness gets across when developed from the Ganda context. The old system, however, has to be adapted in order to regulate present-day problems; one such adaptation would be, for instance, monogamy. The appeal to the traditional moral system would be to its binding nature rather than its content, and the message would still be in accordance with the affective part of the Ganda consciousness, instead of trying to change it.

The message is often weakened by the way the spectators' sense of morality as an instrument of change is used. It is clearly stated promiscuity is immoral behaviour which must be abandoned, while in the same play, the audience is admonished not to regard those people who are already infected as immoral and rather be understanding and sympathetic. The argument "it could happen to all of us" is applied here. Sexual behaviour of people is a sensitive topic, and it is very difficult to change. One can consequently understand the device of the communicators, to refer to moral values as a way to address the issue. In so doing, it is possible to make a case for compassion with the victims of immoral behaviour. The fact that this message very often is modified almost immediately after it is being made, however, weakens it considerably.

To render the AIDS campaign more effective, in Freire's words, more "thematic investigation into people's thinking" is required. Wrong ideas, such as the notion about life expectancy among the Ganda, on the side of the communicators could then be avoided, and the plays would be more relevant.

In addition to the contradictions inherent in the messages of the plays, there are other problems CT against AIDS faces. After four years of information-campaigns, a high awareness among the Ugandan population about channels of infection, methods of transmission, prevention, and protection against AIDS exists, yet there is no indication the rate of infection with AIDS is on the decline - quite the contrary. The campaigns seem to have failed in changing the behaviour of Ugandan society. One of the reasons for this is, that after such a high level of awareness has been achieved, the campaigns should have been taken a step further instead of repeating the same information.[113] In other information campaigns, dealing with the prevention of diseases like measles or whooping cough, there is a follow-up in form of vaccinations. The plays supporting campaigns against those diseases can therefore suggest solutions which can be transformed into reality by the spectators almost immediately without too much effort. This is not possible with AIDS, because there is not yet a vaccine or cure, and also because of the very nature the disease is primarily spread, i.e. sexually transmitted. Maybe the situation should be tackled differently. Since the possibility of vaccination is not there, other follow-ups should be found, and the plays could take a more practical turn. While still conveying information about AIDS and pointing to the social responsibility of all Ugandans to prevent its further spread, they could mention the necessity of testing in order to behave responsibly and not to infect other people. Obviously the playwrights would have to take care that the message would not be diluted. The necessity for a change of behaviour in order to avoid infection, particularly for those people who are not yet infected, would have to come across unmistakably.[114] A report on German TV, for example, about AIDS in Uganda, showed youths of about 14 to 16 years in Rakai District, one of the areas that is worst hit by AIDS. There are villages where only children are left, all the adults having died of AIDS. Older brothers and sisters have now taken over the household tasks and look after the younger children. One young man, about 16 years old, when asked said, that he would like to marry and have children, but that he did not know if he was

[113] To some extent, this is already done by some organisations, like WHO. They have ended the first phase of their campaign, which was mainly intended to spread information about the disease. They have now started their second phase in which they try to modify behaviour in favour of monogamy (conversation with L.B. Wilson, WHO). The problematic nature of this kind of argumentation was discussed earlier on. It should also be noted that, although all NGOs and international organisations advocate "safe sex" and limited sexual relationships/monogamy, there are differences in emphasis. While organisations like UNICEF, Red Cross, EIL, or WHO are primarily interested in the medical aspects of AIDS and therefore promote "safe sex," church and religious NGOs stress the moral aspect of promiscuity.

[114] Free testing is available from all district medical officers. It has to be pointed out that of those Ugandans who went for free testing in downtown Kampala, fewer than 30% came back for the results (L.B. Wilson, WHO). Admittedly, I cannot substantiate the hypothesis that the knowledge of one's HIV-status will positively influence behaviour. This hypothesis does not consider attitudes like those of people who, knowing that they have AIDS, try to make the most of their remaining life by having as many sexual partners as possible; or those of people who try to infect as many others as they can; or those who are convinced that they do not have AIDS and therefore don't have to change their behaviour. I have the impression, however, that those attitudes are the exception. Since the consciousness raising campaigns appeal to the audience's sense of social responsibility, it is, in my opinion, a logical conclusion to suggest more testing.

HIV-positive or not. In the same report, a wedding was shown, and it was mentioned that the couple did not know it's HIV-status. The 'journey' to the nearest town, about five miles away, where they could get tested was out of the question, because the money for the trip could be spend on other urgent needs of the family. Coincidentally, the Church of Uganda and the Catholic Churches in Uganda now require pre-marital blood screening. What the report shows nevertheless is that it is extremely important to follow up on the dissemination of information with measures to give people a chance to find out about their HIV-status and not wait for them to take the initiative. They could then behave accordingly.[115]

I do not mean to imply that no additional information is needed; quite the contrary. Information campaigns are necessary, but with a topic as sensitive as AIDS, the content as well as the form of the messages have to be scrutinised. The contradictions seen in the plays are in fact symptomatic of the nationwide campaign against AIDS, and not just for theatre. An evaluation study carried out by the AIDS Control Programme (ACP) and the World Health Organisation between July and December 1991 points to some of the difficulties in the campaign. The respondents e.g. found radio jingles telling them to abstain from sex absurd.[116] The report also showed that there is a demand for more information, especially about condom use.[117] Resentment of condom use was found to be caused by campaigns of religious leaders against condoms. There is a need for more information, and theatre could be employed effectively for that purpose. Some of the contradictions inherent in the plays will have to be solved outside the theatre as they are social rather than theatrical problems.

After discussing some theoretical aspects occuring in CT, in the next chapter, their application in the plays will be looked at. By now, the AIDS epidemic constitutes a reality in Ugandan society to such an extent that theatre, as other media, cannot but comment on the disease. In the following, various forms of TFD plays dealing with AIDS will be described.

---

115 The report about Rakai district stands in contrast to WHO's information about the district. According to WHO, most people in Rakai have been tested.

116 *Weekly Topic*, March 7, 1992.

117 The report points out that a sizeable number or respondents were found to be not knowledgeable in the use of condoms: in the districts of Mukono, Kabale and Mbale, out of a total of 977 respondents, 35 percent could identify a wrapped condom, 73 per cent had heard about it, and 62 percent knew that it could prevent AIDS; s. *Weekly Topic*, March 7, 1992.

4. CASE STUDIES

4.1. Patterns and Techniques in Campaign Theatre

Before discussing the actual plays, I will present some general thoughts which have to be considered when producing a CT play in the concrete Ugandan setting.

The plays discussed in this chapter, represent a type of TFD that can best be described with the term urban plays to raise consciousness. They are written and created in and around Kampala, and from there are taken up-country. They are primarily informative and concerned with topics like child care, environmental problems, information about immunisation, AIDS education et al. Their aim is to educate people on specific problematic issues. It is assumed the information given in the plays will increase awareness of the fact that people have to modify behaviour in order to solve the respective problem. The plays aim to sensitise target audiences for the recognition of existing problems, for their causes, and also to make them realise solutions can be reached by a change of attitudes and life style.

Primary consideration, therefore, is the effectiveness of a play rather than its aesthetic value; this is not to insinuate that plays have no aesthetic value at all. In *Give A Chance*, for example, the audience obviously enjoyed a mime scene in which AIDS is the personified chairman of the killer diseases.[1] A play that makes the audience laugh has a certain aesthetic quality,[2] but the point that should be stressed, is that it is not the primary concern of a didactic play to provide entertainment and enjoyment. It uses its entertainment quality to convey information to an audience. An educative play has to be entertaining to arouse the interest of the spectators - if the play is boring nobody will hear its message. Plays dealing with a concrete project, on the other hand, stimulate a very different kind of interest. Since these plays are ideally performed by members of the target group, other members of the community are interested to hear what their fellow-villagers have to say. The entertainment arises from that interest. CT, however, is not usually performed by the target group. Inasmuch as the play is supposed to give information which is necessary to create a new attitude

---

1 For a detailed discussion of *Give A Chance* s. chapter 4.4.1.

2 Personal interview with Chris Dunton, Bayreuth, 13/7/91; s.a. aesthetic function of costume and dance, chapter 4.4.1.

in the audience, this information cannot possibly come from within the target group. To arouse interest, the play has to bring its message across through entertainment which is accomplished with the help of music, dance and mime. The opposite of CT is commercial popular urban theatre which deals with the same topics, although not for the purpose of achieving change. To demonstrate this distinction, I have included a sub-chapter on the productions of JK Ebonita, one of the popular urban theatre groups; their plays are designed to entertain. Reference to AIDS is made because the disease constitutes a part in the life of Ugandan society, and is considered of interest to the audience and can therefore be transferred into entertainment.

The techniques and mechanisms of CT become clearer when comparing them to those of the purely project-oriented plays usually performed in rural areas. In order to be effective, i.e. to bring about a change of behaviour, in both plays for raising consciousness as well as in project-oriented plays, it is important to clearly define the problem that needs to be solved. Moreover, it has to become clear to the audience what the development aim is. In project-oriented plays, the discussion of the ways which lead to that aim, the "participatory research to identify the problems, and organise the human, financial, and material resources of the community can be achieved through development theatre activities with relatively little help from outside."[3] Health issues, however, require both knowledge and resources from outside. Breitinger points out that problem analysis and health education should only be carried out by medically trained personnel which are not usually available in the suburban villages and rural areas. And too, serum for vaccination, syringes and disinfectants are not available and cannot be supplied from local resources or administered by local people; the expertise of medical doctors, nurses or health workers is required. In Campaign Theatre, the recipients of the information have to remain passive as far as the purely medical content is concerned: "they can and should, however, be involved in the organisation of the campaigns, in the mobilisation of the audiences, and in follow-up activities. And they should participate in the wider context of general information about health issues."[4] The aims and methods of the campaign must be spelled out clearly to the audience. In all the plays discussed in this chapter, it is made clear that AIDS is spreading fast. The aim is for people to realise that anybody may

3 Breitinger, "Popular Urban Theatre," p. 282.

4 ibid., p. 282.

become infected, and the only way to avoid it is a change in sexual behaviour.

Obviously CT plays will be performed as often as possible so the message can reach large portions of the populace. This is in contrast to plays dealing with a concrete project, as they have only to be performed once in order to solve a certain problem. In Ugandan Campaign Theatre other media, cassettes, video and film, are also used to support live theatre performances when it comes to disseminating the information: Philly Lutaaya gave his message in concerts, and also on his cassette and in a film;[5] international organisations as WHO, Red Cross, EIL produce videos which are then shown on information tours in the villages. Similarly, the Association of Performing Artists in Uganda (APAU) recorded the AIDS Quake Festival and now uses the video for information campaigns in schools. The AIDS Drama Competition for primary schools, where the same play was performed by all primary schools in the country, is the clearest example of the advertising nature of CT: the same information has to reach large numbers of the population.

It is in accordance with their aim of convincing the audience of their message that didactic plays - both project-oriented and CT - do not develop their characters. The characters are presented as types reflecting one particular trait rather than being fully developed individuals. They either stand for one age-group, or different professional groups. Belonging to a specific social group is, in fact, the only trait that distinguishes them. The primary aim of the plays is to show correct behaviour as opposed to the wrong one. The creation of complex, individual personalities involves the risk of spoiling the clarity of the message. To the producers, it is more important to concentrate fully on the one aspect of behaviour to be changed thereby ensuring the audience's attention is focussed. The message as to what is right and what is wrong, is presented unambiguously to avoid possible misunderstandings among the spectators.

In didactic plays, the information is usually conveyed through dialogue with the characters on stage representing the life of the majority of the spectators. Since the characters have so few individual traits, everybody is able to see him- or herself depicted in the play. Equally, their conversations are of the kind that anyone among the audience could have. This similarity

5 Philly Lutaaya was a famous Ugandan pop-star who had declared publicly that he had AIDS.

is further enhanced by the fact that the plays are designed by Ugandans who translate the medical facts into language, images, and metaphors which are relevant to a Ugandan audience.

Didactic theatre is based on the assumption that it is more interesting to watch a play depicting and discussing problems than listening to a lecture on the same topic; a play is more likely to make the spectators draw a connection between what they see on stage and their own life. It influences both cognitive and affective systems of the audience's consciousness, and involves various senses whereas a lecture has a more scientific, objective character and tries to convince the listeners by appeals to the rational part of their consciousness.

Looking at the structure and purpose of the plays discussed in this chapter, it becomes clear that they, quite unlike literary drama, do not rely heavily on scripts, or rather, their scripts are not as elaborate. They concentrate almost exclusively on dialogue. Non-verbal voice qualities, which are usually to be found in the stage-directions, such as gestures, sounds, mime, are virtually not mentioned at all in the text.[6] The playwrights are primarily concerned with writing down all the information in the dialogue, as they want to write scripts that serve the creation of a play on stage rather than aspiring to create a work of literary value. The non-verbal voice qualities applied in the plays are usually not found in stage-directions but are developed by the actors through improvisations during rehearsals; they are consequently in the repertoire but not in the script. Campaign Theatre takes a position between literary drama and TFD plays dealing with a concrete project. Whereas literary drama usually has an elaborate, carefully worked out script, with extensive stage-directions, project-oriented plays have no script at all. The idea for such plays comes from the target group who creates the plays through improvisations during rehearsals. In Campaign Theatre, in order to avoid misunderstandings among the audience and the possible spread of inaccurate messages, the factual information about AIDS has to be in the script and cannot be changed by improvisations. Only some room is left for improvising when performance techniques, such as body-language and gestures, are concerned, but the scripts are specific about which songs and which music is

6 s.a. the discussion of para-language in Fernando Poyatos, *New Perspectives in Nonverbal Communication. Studies in Cultural Anthropology, Social Psychology, Linguistics, Literature, and Semiotics* (Oxford, New York, Toronto, Sydney, Paris, Frankfurt: Pergamon Press, 1983), p. 327.

to be played. This is in accordance with the very nature of CT which involves the target group only to a limited degree. International organisations and NGOs provide funding and information - all of which is translated into the Ugandan context by the playwrights who write the scripts. Those scripts in turn are given to the various theatrical groups who perform them without any alterations. Artistic interpretation of the plays' content is not desired. On the contrary, the scripts are supposed to make sure the messages reaching the various audiences are identical.

4.1.1. Language, Site, and Mood

A problem with didactic plays in Uganda is language. Uganda consists of different ethnic groups which speak different languages. This has to be considered by producers of plays that are supposed to be shown in different parts of the country, since each "language possesses some distinctive attributes of its own which also must be known before an outsider can hope to communicate effectively or before an observer can evolve categories for a valid analysis."[7] Also, each language has taboo-words which should be known by the playwrights so they can avoid using them and thereby avoid offending the audience. Finally, the vocabulary of a language may have certain deficiencies, for example there may be no words for certain objects, actions, or ideas.[8] Usually, in these cases, the missing word is substituted either by direct translation from another language or by just accepting a foreign word or expression. In the Ugandan AIDS campaign, for instance, there are two slogans which appear in every play about AIDS: "zero grazing" and "love carefully." These slogans are so widely known by now that in all probability, they will always remain in English, no matter in which language the play is performed.

An important insight is the fact that languages reflect people's mode of acquiring knowledge, and therefore, also affect prevalent modes of communicating information about such knowledge.[9] A play is accordingly most effective, when it is created by people who speak the language. This is done only to a limited extent in Ugandan TFD where the plays are in English rather than in Ugandan languages. This is partly due to the involvement of international organisations, and partly to the fact that the

---

7 Doob, *Communication in Africa*, p. 190.

8 ibid., p. 196.

9 ibid., p. 197.

plays discussed here were written and created by artists in Kampala where people from all over the country, from different ethnic groups, as well as foreigners and expatriates live and work. The language that enables them to communicate is English and most people therefore have some knowledge of it. In most of the areas up-country, however, people do not speak English. It would be difficult for them to follow a play when shown on TV or on video. One way to avoid that kind of problem would be to no longer have the plays come from the centre Kampala, but to create them regionally and produce them in different languages, according to the region where they are performed. Another possibility would be to reduce dialogue and, instead, put the stress on mime, gesture and music.[10] The short mime-scene in *Give A Chance*, in which the infection with HIV was enacted visually, was understood by everybody.

Whether a play is regarded as pure entertainment or as informative, depends not only on the message conveyed through language, but on the site where it is performed. A play that is performed at the National Theatre, for example, will encourage less audience participation than a play performed at a central place in a village. The site of the National Theatre makes the audience behave according to European theatre 'rules,' i.e., to sit passively and watch.[11] In a village, the environment is familiar from village meetings and discussions and is not connected with passivity; spectators in a village setting usually know each other and are not shy to talk and make comments. The size of the audience plays an important role in this respect as it can determine the effectiveness of communication.[12]

Various characteristics of the site can determine the size of the audience, one being the location of the site: is the play performed in the market place or in a meeting house which can accommodate a limited number of people? Geographical accessibility affects not only the communicator but also the audience size: how far do people have to travel

[10] This is done by one of the TFD-groups in Nigeria. The actors' way of applying the art of mime, body language, dance and music makes the plays both fascinating to watch as well as easily comprehensible. The group is thereby able to perform plays for a multi-ethnical and multi-lingual audience in markets or taxi-parks in the cities of Nigeria, with most of the spectators understanding the action. In two of the Ugandan plays discussed in this chapter, *Give A Chance* and *Abajambula mu Lubiiri*, that device also was applied (for a detailed discussion, s. chapter 4.4.1.).

[11] The National Theatre at Kampala was built by the British in 1959.

[12] Doob, *Communication in Africa*, p. 123.

to a particular site, and how much effort does it take them?[13] Many people may not be able to spend money for transport to a site where a play is performed. Therefore, to be effective, TFD has to go to the people and not vice versa. Thus in Southern Uganda people are likely to be quite well informed about AIDS, because this is the area where most plays are performed and where people have access to TV, radio, and a greater variety of newspapers. This is not so much the case in the north with its areas of rebel activity and bad roads. The same people, therefore, receive more and more information about AIDS, whereas people in the north hear comparatively little about it.

Not only geographical, but also social accessibility may influence the size of the audience: which rules and regulations enable some people and not others to attend a play? People from the slum areas in Kampala for example are not likely to attend a play at the National Theatre. Likewise, somebody who can afford the entrance fee for the National Theatre will probably not watch a TFD play in a slum area. If a play is performed in a rural area, e.g. in a meeting house, there may be a similar problem: is it, for instance, acceptable for women to go there, or just as important, for children who also have to be educated on AIDS? Especially for outside communicators, like the American NGO *The Experiment in International Living* who go to villages and show their videos, it is important to have some knowledge about social accessibility to reach the target group.

The site at which a communication is received affects the composition of the audience, and it may also influence interaction between the communicator and the audience. First, there are the mechanical aspects of the site, acoustics, distance between communicator and audience, illumination, comfort (heat, cold), protection from rain or sun, seating arrangements, devices (platform rostrum, audio-visual aids), aesthetic qualities.[14] The setting in Lugogo-stadium in Kampala, for example, where the AIDS Quake Festival was held, is not ideal to communicate effectively: the stage was too removed from the audience, so that it was very difficult to understand the words of the play, and the seating arrangement did not encourage audience participation.

The fact the site at which a play is performed may influence the attitude of the audience could explain why many TFD plays are understood

13 ibid., p. 125.

14 ibid., p. 134.

as entertainment rather than informational. To make the plays effective, the communicators must perform them at sites used for communication anyway, like meeting houses, schools, markets et al.

Other aspects influencing the mood of the audience are temporal ones. First is the actual length of a play which must be adapted to the audience's attention span. When trying to determine the ideal length, the attitude towards time of the target group has to be taken into account. Redundancy may cause boredom in one culture whereas it is acceptable in another.[15] In the Ugandan context, a play must not be too short. People who go to the theatre on Sunday afternoons, for example, want to be entertained all afternoon, and not just for an hour or two. Plays in theatre halls ordinarily last three to four hours. Therefore, it is more acceptable in TFD plays to repeat one message on different levels than merely state the problem, give the information and finish the play.

4.1.2. Changes

With both, plays for consciousness raising and project-oriented plays, the post-performance discussion is of utmost importance. The audience has an opportunity to ask questions, speak about what it has just seen, consider new attitudes and a corresponding change of behaviour. Not all the plays discussed in this chapter, however, had a post-performance discussion. It is obvious that plays which are shown on TV, like *It's Not Easy* and *Burdens Of Youth,* cannot have one. Similarly, the AIDS Quake Festival which took place in a gymnasium was not the right forum for discussions. When these plays are taken up-country or to schools as videos, however, they are used to stimulate conversations. Philly Lutaaya took every opportunity to speak with people during his campaign, so they could ask questions and talk freely with him.

In conclusion, it must be reiterated that communication aimed at changing behaviour has to be reinforced to be effective. The message has to be repeated often so the spectators eventually internalise it. Doob argues that repetition can be very helpful as it may increase the probability of perception, comprehension, and retention.[16] He warns however, that it may also cause boredom in the audience if applied too often. In Ganda culture,

---

15 ibid. p. 236.

16 Doob, p. 229.

repetition is an important feature which can be found everywhere: in music, story-telling, conversation. The greeting, for example, is not only uttered once when two or more persons meet; it will be repeated at more or less regular intervals during a conversation. It is, consequently, reasonable to expect Baganda to react favourably to repetitions in a play.[17]

4.2. Theatre against AIDS

Having discussed practical factors to be taken into account when producing a didactic play, I now present examples depicting various ways of dealing with AIDS through theatre. I have included a sub-chapter discussing the productions of the popular urban theatre group JK Ebonita although I would not classify their plays as TFD. Their work is discussed in this study for two reasons. Firstly, by contrasting it to TFD, it helps to demonstrate the relationship between entertainment and education in Campaign Theatre, and secondly, JK Ebonita's approach to the topic AIDS is an example for a theatrical way of dealing with the disease that differs from TFD, which is performed primarily for the purpose of education. The primary concern of artists who produce popular urban comedies is having sold out shows, rather than to facilitate discussions about AIDS; they want to entertain, and they try to address issues of concern to a wide cross section of society. Problems such as bad hospital conditions, corrupt policemen, etc., are critically exposed, but the criticism is presented in such a way so as not to make the audience feel uneasy. *The Dollar* by JK Ebonita exemplifies this kind of play. It is a crime story about a husband who goes to the police station to report his wife missing. Eventually, it turns out that he himself has killed her in order to get her money. The play lasts about three and a half hours and mixed with the plot of the crime story, are musical interludes and episodes dealing with topical issues. The first scene e.g. comically depicts a day at a police station. In a satirical way, the scene lays open the degree of corruption among policemen: those people with money to pay bribes are either not punished for their crimes or get better treatment. A lawyer who is imprisoned is still able to lead a comfortable life in his cell, with his girl-friends visiting him and bringing him food. The scene also depicts a landlord coming in with his housegirl and accusing her of theft, whereas the girl complains about sexual harrassment. The landlord bribes one of the

[17] Domestic comedies, the most popular genre in Ugandan theatre, are also built around a pattern of repetitions. In those 3 to 4 hour long plays, jokes and episodes are repeated with only slight variations - with the audience obviously enjoying it.

policemen, which settles the matter in his favour. The episode is presented in a comical manner which typifies that kind of play. The audience probably has had annoying experiences with corrupt policemen and can identify with what is criticised in the play. The criticism, however, is made in a general way so the problem is exposed but no actions or solutions are proposed. The audience has the feeling its problems are depicted in the play. By ridiculing the problem, producers take care that the spectators are not too upset. As Breitinger remarks, "the attraction of this kind of theatre seems to lie in its combination of fanciful fabrications with the laughing away of social malpractices."[18] The play is, after all, supposed to entertain. Reference to AIDS in those plays is made similarly in that it never constitutes the dominant topic. As with other problems, AIDS is mentioned in only one episode, very often in a light-hearted, funny way as in the last scene of *The Dollar*. The play ends with a scene in the departure hall at Entebbe Airport where a long queue is waiting to check in. In the queue a young man is trying to make a pass at young ladies. He fails a few times until one of the women behind him responds to his questions and speaks to him. She tells him that she is on her way to the U.K. for medical treatment. He, quite happy about his apparent success with her, asks what her problem is, to which she replies "AIDS." The audience is amused at the young man's apparent ill luck. The reference to AIDS here is made in a very comical way. The purpose obviously is not to educate the audience about certain aspects of the disease. No factual information is given. AIDS is merely mentioned and used as subject for a joke. A play like *The Dollar* can hardly be classified as TFD. It is a popular urban drama designed to entertain, whereas TFD plays are created for the purpose of education with entertainment as a secondary goal in the service of the didactic purpose.[19]

4.3. Popular Urban Theatre - JK Ebonita

Between 1987 and 1991, a number of urban theatre groups has emerged in Kampala whose plays are extraordinaryly popular with city audiences and who play to capacity audiences.[20] They attract fairly affluent audiences who

---

[18] Breitinger, "Popular Urban Theatre," p. 278.

[19] for further reference s. Breitinger, "Popular Urban Theatre."

[20] Except for JK Ebonita/Jimmy Katumba & the Ebonies, those groups are non-professional. The actors, who during the day have jobs like office-clerks, civil servants, etc., meet only in the evenings for rehearsals. The plays last between three

can afford going to the theatre with the aim of spending an entertaining, agreeable afternoon or evening.[21] In catering to these audiences, the urban theatre groups produce social comedies which address problems of society in a light-hearted, comical way, combined with mild social criticism. Audiences can identify with the critical attitude adopted in the play but not feel offended.

One of the most popular theatre groups in Kampala is JK Ebonita. The group is part of Jimmy Katumba & the Ebonies, a noted Ugandan pop-group. They perform every weekend at the Theatre Excelsior in Kampala which has a seating capacity of 700 to 1000 spectators, regularly selling out their plays and music shows. One reason for their popularity is that they are bi-lingual; actors switch back and forth between English and Luganda thereby enabling both Luganda- and non-Luganda speakers to follow the plot. The audience at the Theatre Excelsior, consequently, consists of both Ugandans and expatriates.[22] In addition to catering to a mixed audience, JK Ebonita tries to address as many Ugandans as possible. The long duration of the plays allows for the integration of unrelated episodes and songs into the main plot. These episodes critically address issues that play a role in Ugandan society, as e.g AIDS. As exemplified in the last scene of *The Dollar*, "all these malpractices are presented rather off-handedly, as if more for comic effect than as serious criticism."[23] This element of social commitment is balanced by musical interludes in which the popular songs of Jimmy Katumba are played, giving the band an opportunity to show off sophisticated technology like synthesizers and video equipment. The songs are usually accompanied by dances mixing elements of folk-dance with modern disco-dancing. This combination is also reflected in the costumes: some dancers wear traditional Baganda dancing costumes, whereas others are dressed in Western-style disco-fashion. By wearing the traditional Baganda costume on stage, the group tries to appeal to the Ugandans among the audience on an emotional level. In an examination of the

---

and four hours and are performed on weekends, both in the afternoon and in the evening.

21 The audience typically includes businessmen, traders, consultants, the newly-rich merchants, sometimes students who happen to have free tickets.

22 The Excelsior gives consultants, development-workers and other foreigners an opportunity to attend plays; most of the other plays performed in Kampala are in Luganda - with the exception of one English show every three months at the National Theatre.

23 Breitinger, "Popular Urban Theatre," p. 276.

function of clothing, Bogatyrev has analysed costume as a sign system linking the wearer with certain social groupings or attitudes.[24] Winner describes Bogatyrev's view of functions as "special aims fulfilled by the costume which transform these costumes from simple use objects (...) to signs which function much in the same way that verbal signs do, and in which there is, as in all semiotic acts, a multitude of functions, and thus of meanings."[25] Thus costumes may function as signs of social or economic differentiation, of nationality, of occupation etc. In the case of members of Ebonita/Ebonies, wearing the traditional Baganda dancing costume, has the function of marking it as 'our costume' - a function called by Bogatyrev "the function of the structure of functions."[26] He sees the function of 'our costume' as similar to that of the regionalistic or nationalistic function, but there is a fundamental difference between them: "Whereas a costume with a dominant regionalistic function will be placed categorically in opposition to costumes of other regions, 'our costume' is close to its wearers and lacks this sense of opposition."[27] The function of 'our costume' clearly has an emotional coloring. Seeing its traditional dancing costume on stage is supposed to give the audience a feeling of belonging. This device is also repeated on the level of music and dance. Although the dance-songs have modern lyrics they use the rhythm of traditional songs. The dances include characteristic movements of traditional dances, particularly the shaking of the hips, although these too are combined with disco-dance elements. Dance is a non-verbal method of communication, and as such, an important part of culture: with and through dance, ideas, knowledge, cultural values, social relationships and activities, religious believes, emotions, poetics et al. can be expressed.[28] According to Giurchescu, dance obtains semantic meaning through its function determined by the socio-cultural context.[29] Dance does not exist as independent language within cultural communication. It acquires meaning through its relationship to the other

---

24 Bogatyrev, *The Functions of Folk Costume in Moravian Slovakia* (The Hague, Paris: Mouton, 1971); s.a. discussion of Bogatyrev's study in T. Winner, "Some Fundamental Concepts," p. 80.

25 Bogatyrev, *The Functions of Folk Costume*, p. 93; T. Winner, "Some Fundamental Concepts," p. 80.

26 Bogatyrev, p. 96; s.a. T. Winner, p. 80.

27 Bogatyrev, p. 96.

28 Weidig, *Tanz-Ethnologie*, p. 82/3.

29 Anca Giurchescu, "La danse comme object sémiotique," p. 176, in Weidig, *Tanz-Ethnologie*, p. 71.

types of communication.[30] Dance as a reflection of culture cannot be understood as independent from the other elements of that culture, only as an integrated part of it. In the case of Ebonita, presenting traditional dances mixed with disco-elements, the dances no longer have their original function. What used to be war- and wedding-dances, or dances for certain festivities, are now deprived of their content by transferral onto a proscenium stage, where they lack one of their most distinctive feature, i.e. the participation of community members. By performing on stage, in front of a passive audience, the dances are no longer alive as elements of Ganda culture, only their outward appearance, the familiar movements, are still there. Desai remarks that what originated as a popular theatrical form becomes de-popularized through the process of urban appropriation: "Although it bears a certain formal resemblance to its original source, the appropriate performance ceases to be a site of popular articulation and moves away from the processual discursive practice of popular theatre and towards a different discursive practice."[31] They now function as reminders of Ganda culture rather than representative elements. It is doubtful if they have any other effect, apart from pure entertainment.

The combination of traditional Baganda elements, eg. costume, dance, music, with those of Western culture serves several purposes. The function of urban/Western dress differs considerably from that of folk costume.[32] It is associated with progress, modernity, and open-mindedness. By displaying some of the attributes of Western culture, disco-rhythms, -dress, -dance, on stage, a link is made between values and customs of traditional Ganda society and progress which is associated with the West. The audience has the impression of getting the best of both worlds: it is reassured that in the course of development it has not ignored its cultural roots, while at the same time the notion of progress is conveyed. On another level, the combination of 'our costume' and 'Western costume,' of 'our dance' and 'disco dance,' has to be seen within the context of Ebonita's/Ebonies' plays. With their combination of crime story, social criticism, and music show, JK Ebonita appeal to various social and professional groups in Unganda: intellectuals, businessmen, market-people/traders, people from rural as well as urban areas, old and young people.

---

30 Weidig, *Tanz-Ethnologie*, p. 70/1.

31 Desai, "Theater as Praxis," p. 68.

32 Bogatyrev, *The Functions of Folk Costume*, p. 97.

For a Festival on World AIDS Day 1989 in Kampala, JK Ebonita contributed a video-clip with a short play on AIDS: in front of a disco, a young man, Moses, waits for his girl-friend. He falls asleep and has a dream in which he dances with prostitutes at the disco. At the end of the evening, he leaves the place with three women. The next scene - still part of his dream - is set in the village. Moses comes home, very thin, coughing, with a skin disease and stomach pain, typical symptoms of AIDS. In the background, the three women from the disco can be seen watching in disbelief. Moses' mother tries to help him by calling a traditional healer to treat him. After the healer has left, Moses falls asleep and dreams of a mask dancing around him, singing "Love more carefully," one of Jimmy Katumba's popular hits. Then the scene shifts back: Moses wakes up in front of the disco as his girl-friend arrives, two hours late. He realises that he only suffered from AIDS in the dream. He and his girl-friend enter the disco where the pop-star Jimmy Katumba is just interrupting his performance for the interval. Still remembering his dream, Moses steps on stage and sings a song: "Love more carefully."

The video-clip conveys the message that AIDS is caused by promiscuity, by opposing city-life with all the dangers of its glamorous nightlife and village life with its traditional value system. Only when the healer cannot help him anymore, Moses realises the importance of adhering to traditional moral values. The contradiction is resolved in the end, when Moses wakes up and realises that he has only been dreaming. In reality, he has only one girl-friend, and the message is that he and his girl-friend are both faithful and therefore not in danger of contracting AIDS. In the song at the end of the video-clip, "Love more carefully," the importance of this kind of monogamous life-style is re-emphasized. By presenting village-life with its intact value system as solution while at the same time advocating monogamy, the message becomes ambigious, since the Ganda moral system allows for polygamy. It becomes obvious here, that two aspects have to be distinguished in plays for AIDS education. On the one hand, there is the technical aspect of using elements of Ganda culture in order to appeal to the audience. On the other hand, the culture has to be infiltrated with foreign ideas like monogamy, in order to convey the message that only a change of behaviour can stop the spread of AIDS.

The message of the video-clip is weakened by a contradiction developing from the costumes. On the one hand, the suggested solution is a return to traditional Ganda moral norms which is implied visually by contrasting city-life, where Moses caught AIDS, and village-life, where he goes to for comfort, once he is sick. On the other hand, in the last scene the importance of monogamy is demonstrated by showing Moses as having only one girl-friend. As a result, a contradiction develops between the cognitive, rational system of the audience that understands the demand for monogamy and faithfulness in order to avoid the infection with AIDS; and its affective, subconscious system. On that level, an appeal is made to traditional moral norms with visual elements belonging to Western culture. The communication thus works only on a very superficial level which may not result in a change of behaviour.

The main purpose of the video-clip is entertainment. The actor who plays Moses, is one of Ebonita's best dancers, and in the disco-scene he has ample opportunity to show his skill. Then, there is the dancing mask which, with its elaborate costume, is also fascinating to watch. The other actors on stage are dressed in rather disco-like fashion. To a Ugandan audience, these costumes are appealing in themselves for after 20 years of almost complete isolation from the developments of international show-business, they now see elements of Western pop-culture on stage. With their elaborate costumes and sound equipment, JK Ebonita in a way take the place that film and TV have in Western culture. This is also reflected in the design of their plays. The montage of motives, themes and structural elements imitates that of foreign TV serials, broadcast by Radio Uganda, as Breitinger also remarks: "The influence of television dramaturgy is pervasive, alike in plot development, in scenic structure and design, and even in the lavishness and frequency of the costume changes, particularly among the female protagonists."[33] Obviously, what is important in their video-clip, is the performance rather than the topic AIDS.

In the group's play, *The Wedshock,* Ebonita introduces a song about AIDS. In typical concert fashion, the song, sung in Luganda, is not really integrated into the plot. It portrays the dangers of AIDS in a humorous way. During the song, condoms are distributed on stage; this has a rather comical effect on the audience. Obviously, it is not intended to provoke serious discussions about AIDS, and it is not the main topic of the play. It is introduced because condom use is hotly debated in Ugandan society. The spectators see their problems being addressed on stage, but the presentation is such that it is possible to laugh them off. No new information about the

---

33 Breitinger, "Popular Urban Theatre," p. 276.

disease is conveyed to the audience. Whereas after 'real' TFD plays about AIDS, condoms are frequently distributed, the distribution of condoms on stage, among the actors in *The Wedshock* only serves the purpose of entertainment.

JK Ebonita's way of presenting AIDS through theatre exemplifies the approach of the popular commercial theatre groups. Contrary to TFD, they do not attempt to depict characters and situations on stage with whom the audience can easily identify. The atmosphere and social images presented in the plays are not those of the majority of the Ugandan population, "it lies far beyond the social realities of the spectators, but appears to be within the range of their fanciful aspirations."[34] The cheating and murdering of the affluent characters on stage is so far removed from the social reality of the spectators they do not see any relevance to their own lives. The main purpose for dealing with the disease is to attract large audiences. It is in accordance with that aim to adopt subject-matters of TFD, like AIDS, because AIDS is an "in"-topic. It is here, however, where the parallels between TFD and popular urban theatre stop. Since the over-all aim of a group like JK Ebonita is commercial, they employ theatrical techniques primarily because of their entertainment character. As seen in the group's video-clip, folk-dance and costume are presented in a way that suggests a synthesis of Ganda culture with that of the West rather than a return to a strict value system.[35]

Having discussed the approach of a commercially oriented theatre group towards AIDS, I now describe various CT projects which were designed to spread information about AIDS.

4.4. CT Plays Sponsored by International Organisations

International organisations recognise the usefulness of theatre as a means for disseminating information and work with Ugandan artists to further AIDS education. In the following two sub-chapters, two projects, one financed by WHO and the other one by UNICEF, will be discussed. They differ in the manner they approach the theatrical aspect of the projects. On the organisational level, however, they apply the same method; both projects are carried out in close cooperation with indigenous

---

34 ibid., p. 277.

35 s. Desai on the de-popularization of dance and costume, p. 55 of this work.

organisations.[36] It is hoped that these TFD plays will, through their use of theatrical techniques and metaphors, manage to relate to Ugandan society rather than to impose foreign ways of communication. The World Health Organisation (WHO), for example, financed the AIDS Quake Festival which was carried out by the Association of Performing Artists in Uganda (APAU), and UNICEF sponsored a drama-competition which was organised jointly by the Ministry of Education and Ugandan artists. The competition was judged by a committee of Ugandans who work in the field of theatre, like Prof. Rose Mbowa from the Department of Music, Dance and Drama (MDD) at Makerere University, Mary Jane Musungu from the National Theatre, Peter Lwanga from JK Ebonita, et al.

4.4.1. AIDS Quake - Workshop and Festival

In 1989, APAU began a public awareness campaign on AIDS, utilizing theatre. The campaign, called "AIDS Quake - Artists Against AIDS," was sponsored by the AIDS Control Programme and WHO and culminated in a concert on World AIDS Day, December 1st, to educate the general public on the origin, spread, prevention and control of AIDS. To provide the artists with adequate information, a three-day work-shop was held at the National Theatre in Kampala, assisted by the National AIDS Control Programme which handled the AIDS education. The workshop wanted to give "accurate technical information required to embark on an active campaign on the prevention, control and elimination of stigmatization of AIDS."[37] It also attempted to identify critical AIDS themes that are crucial for AIDS prevention. Additionally, it was intended to "develop a detailed plan for action on specific strategies to be adopted by various sectors of APAU, i.e. musicians, dramatists, poets in preparation for AIDS Quake," and to "ensure the continued support, commitment and participation of APAU after AIDS Quake."[38] The workshop was attended by a cross section of artists, freelance writers, musicians, dramatists, poets, graphic and visual artists, band leaders, school teachers, University and secondary school students, popular bands, drama and singing groups.[39] It gave a scientific,

---

[36] The fact that one of the projects was launched in 1989 and the other one in 1991 accounts for some of the differences.

[37] *A Report on APAU Workshop*. 25th - 27th September, 1989. IEC - ACP.

[38] ibid.

[39] ibid.

global and national overview of AIDS and tried to cover most of its crucial aspects, such as origin and cause, socio-economic implications, misconceptions and common questions, prevention and control, facts about condom use, cultural habits that promote the spread of AIDS (tatooing, the custom of blood-brotherhood, circumcision etc.), identifying and addressing target groups, effective communication skills in presenting the AIDS message, and patient care.

The workshop began with a pretest to estimate the level of knowledge about AIDS and ended with a similar test. Although the initial level of knowledge among the participants was high, it was found to have improved by the end of the three days.[40] The workshop consisted of both group-work by the participants as well as lectures. The artists split into four groups to identify their expectations of the seminar. The same was done when it came to the discussion of cultural habits that promote the spread of AIDS in Uganda. Even though communication between the organisers and participants of the workshop appeared to be symmetric with all of them developing insights together, the relationship, in fact, was asymmetric since the implication that there are cultural practices which enhance the risk of infection was made by the organisers of the workshop.[41] Lectures were given when required for a scientific global overview over the disease, its social-economic implications and medical facts. By the end of the workshop, the dramatists among the participants had decided to produce a play for World AIDS Day.

The participants were given to understand entries could be in a language of the contributor's choice. Only material that had never been broadcast, telecast, printed, published, exhibited or demonstrated was accepted. Funds raised from the activities were to benefit AIDS victims and orphans, participating members and APAU.

On World AIDS Day 1989, the artists had the opportunity to present their program in the Festival held in a gymnasium at Lugogo/ Kampala; that Lugogo is a gymnasium and not a theatre hall, illustrated some inherent disadvantages. The acoustics in the hall were inadequate, and while this did not matter too much for the musical performances, the plays were

---

40 ibid.

41 It should be noted that this is a didactic situation not unique for Uganda. The device of disguising an asymmetric relationship as symmetric is applied in workshops all over the world. The participants are challenged to develop results rather than absorbing information passively.

difficult to hear and understand. Additionally, the distance between stage and audience proved to be too great. The middle-section of the hall, usually the place for ball games, was not used for seats; spectators instead were seated on rising bleacher seats at the fringe of the pitch. This arrangement created a separation between stage and audience unsuited for the purpose. Discussions or direct interaction between audience and actors, which is crucial for the project oriented TFD plays, was not possible, and maybe not intended by the organisers. The Festival had the character of an entertainment show with the audience passively watching.

Besides songs, poems and dramatic sketches, two longer plays were shown during the three days of the Festival. One of them, *Give A Chance*, was written by the actor and playwright David Kateete. It begins whith somebody carrying a poster across the stage on which is written "During the year 2029," followed by another poster saying "Sorry, that is a mistake, it is 1989," thus leaving no doubt that the problems which are to be presented on stage concern the Ugandan society at the present time. The main characters are a young girl and an old man with the representative names of Five-Fourteen and Oldpa. The first two scenes consist of dialogues between Five-Fourteen and Oldpa. Scene 1 serves as exposition presenting the problem, introducing the characters, and explaining that in the aftermath of the AIDS Quake, when AIDS has destroyed life like an earthquake, all people, except Five-Fourteen and Oldpa, have died of AIDS. Those age groups, as the sexually inactive groups, are the only ones not affected by the AIDS-catastrophe. In Scene 2, Five-Fourteen wants to know why all the other people have died, and Oldpa tries to explain:

5-14: Isn't this why all those people were contaminated? All those from 15-25 years to whom sexmating was a shortlived pleasure, wild and purposeless? All those from there to 40 to whom sexmating was so sweet and only remedy after the troubles of the day? And those above 40 who had to have a good time before retiring?

Oldpa: You have said it again. That is why you are free 5-14. That is why you have to be protected very preservatively. You are the only light of hope for mankind.[42]

The play tries to show that AIDS can only be conquered through education and information. It is very important therefore, to make this information

42 David Kateete, *Give A Chance*, unpublished play, 1989. p. 8.

available to the children, for it is their generation that can be saved from AIDS:

5-14:	Look at yourself Oldpa. Right now, you are standing for all the grownups. The parents who misguide their off-spring... That is how you grownups want us to stay. Half-knowledged. Yet we don't want to be kept in the dark... We clumsily start venturing into the secret lands where the sweet apple fruit yields in abundance...

The issue of the hierarchical nature of Ganda-society, which does not encourage children to ask questions, is critically addressed here. It is conveyed that this behaviour has to change. Children must be encouraged to ask questions, and they have to be enlightened on sexual matters in order to have a chance to avoid infection with HIV. During the course of the play, concepts such as "safe sex" and "zero grazing" are explained and discussed. 5-14 asks questions, just as other children of her age would probably like to ask, but either do not dare ask their parents, or do not get any answers from them.[43] A relationship between parents and children is thus demonstrated and suggested that is not known in Ganda-society: when children ask questions, claiming their right for information. Oldpa tries to answer these questions. Frequently, he is embarassed and tries to be evasive, but Five-Fourteen keeps on asking. It is unmistakable that eventhough it may be difficult and against the behaviour usually adopted towards children, there has to be dialogue. Children have a right to gather all the information necessary to know how to protect themselves. Oldpa's explanations are livened up by contradictions and interruptions from Five-Fourteen:

5-14:	A crime so big that you are talking about stopping what God himself started. The only aspect of life that makes it worth a living. There had to be some other ways.
Oldpa:	There were other ways, of course...
5-14:	Oh! Surely?! What were these?
Oldpa:	Safe sex, for example.[44]

Scene 2 ends with the appearance of a young man, and all three characters fall into a freeze. The development of the disease AIDS is then enacted in a mime scene. Killer diseases like whooping cough, measles, diarrhoea are personified. The actors representing the killer diseases wear tight gymnastic

43 This also emphasises the need for more information, since the refusal of parents to answer those questions may not only have to do with the traditional attitude of discouraging questions by children, but also with not knowing the right answers. The reference to tradition may be a convenient excuse in this case.

44 *Give A Chance*, p. 13.

suits and banners with their names on it. Through music, dance and mime, it is conveyed that the diseases are holding a conference with AIDS as their chairman. The infection with AIDS is visualized by healthy people dancing with those who are already infected, then falling to the ground, and afterwards carrying a banner with the inscription "AIDS CASE." Dance here is used as a symbol for sexual intercourse, which is underscored by the tight gymnastic suits of the personified diseases, serving an erotic function, the goal being to attract attention.[45] Bogatyrev gives the example of a girl making an effort to attract the attention of a young man by dressing up, to show that the aesthetic and the erotic function of costume may coincide, as is the case with the personified diseases. The aesthetic function of the costume aims at the audience, whereas its erotic function works within the play itself. The apparent attractiveness of the personified Chairman AIDS is taken as a metaphor for the temptation of sexual pleasure. That this pleasure only lasts for a very short time and leads to disease is shown in the dance, when those people who have not resisted the temptation and danced with AIDS, become HIV-carriers. When HIV tries to dance with Five-Fourteen, the young man attacks and, eventually, beats him.[46] HIV flees; AIDS has been defeated by the new generation, which has adhered to the principle of fidelity. It therefore "met the conditions to become a new original parent couple after the visitation of humankind by AIDS, a new original parent couple as Noah and his wife after the flood."[47]

The play ends with an epilogue. A new generation is born which is free of AIDS, the children of Five-Fourteen and the young man. Oldpa is dying and once more, he admonishes everybody to stick to moral values. The play ends on an optimistic note, with everybody singing the title song:

ALL: We are here the future generation
That's free of AIDS
We want to see all the sons of creation
AIDS free
Give a Chance to the Children of today
To make a future world without AIDS.

45 s.a. Bogatyrev, "The Erotic Function of Costume," in *The Function of Folk Costume*, p. 75-77.

46 The way dance is applied here, clearly stands in contrast to how it is done in Ebonita's shows. Whereas Ebonita deprives traditional folk dance of its meaning and uses it as entertainment, in *Give A Chance*, a new dance is created with the aim to communicate a message to the audience.

47 Breitinger, "Popular Urban Theatre," p. 286.

The play was performed on a simple stage in the big gymnasium in Lugogo. There were no props, and during the two longer scenes, only the main-characters, Five-Fourteen and Oldpa, were on stage, acting in such an intense way that, despite the bad acoustics in the hall, the audience was spell-bound and obviously tried very hard to understand the words.

In *Give A Chance*, the basic facts of AIDS are conveyed through dialogue, thus appealing to the cognitive part of the audience's consciousness. The play, however, does not only work on the rational level. There are also stimulants that trigger the conscientisation on the affective level. In a society like Uganda, where children are of utmost importance, the presentation of a child as the only survivor of the AIDS Quake, has instant appeal. On the one hand, the spectators feel pity for the child, who now has to live with the only other survivor, an old man. On the other hand, it also appeals to the principle of human continuity and vitality - one of the three basic principles of the Ganda moral value system.[48] According to this principle, the continuation of humankind has to be ensured through procreation and children. It is the duty of each member of society to contribute to that continuation. By depicting a child as one of the (as it seems before the appearance of the young man) two survivors of the AIDS-epidemic, an appeal is made to the audience's sense of social responsibility. The only other survivor, an old person, appeals in a different way. Traditionally, old people in Ganda society are treated with respect, being closest to the spirits. Due to their experience, what they say is accepted. Because of this, the admonitions of Oldpa to lead a more moral life, have great authority. Together the two characters, old man and young girl, make the audience accept facts and admonitions about the disease. The play aims to convey the facts about AIDS to the audience by getting it emotionally involved in the fate of the young girl, and by relying on an old man appealing to its traditional value system. People are supposed to realise that they have to change their behaviour in order to create a future for the children. The reference to their traditional identity is re-inforced by the costumes of Oldpa and Five-Fourteen: the old man wears a traditional garment, a 'kansu,'[49] whereas the girl wears a 'kikoye.'[50] Those costumes

48 s. chapter 3.6.3.

49 A 'Kansu' is a long, kaftan-like white garment worn by Ganda men.

50 A 'Kikoye' is a colourful wrapper, usually in the colours red and yellow. Ganda women wear it underneath their traditional 'Busuti' (a long dress with a wide skirt).

clearly serve the function of 'our costume,' emphasising again the concept of social responsibility.[51]

The play identifies promiscuity, irresponsibility, and moral degeneration as causes of the AIDS-catastrophe. A solution is suggested: lead a moral life, i.e. be faithful to one partner. As in JK Ebonita's video clip, the return to the correct traditional moral behaviour is connected to monogamy whereas the traditional acceptance of polygamy is not mentioned at all. That solution is presented visually at the end of the play when a new AIDS-free generation is born as a result of Five-Fourteen's and the young man's moral life style. The appeal to morality in this play is made similarly as in JK Ebonita's video-clip. A return to the strict moral system of the Baganda is suggested, while at the same time the importance of monogamy is stressed. This is based on the notion that, considering the fast spread of AIDS, only a consequent acceptance of monogamy can help. Polygamy, by contrast, is not as safe. It only qualifies as safe sexual behaviour as long as every member of the polygamous household is faithful. Obviously, the more people are involved in a marriage, the more difficult it is to control their sexual behaviour. Although a monogamous relationship is not part of tradition, Ganda culture is still invoked as an instrument to convince the audience to abandon both prostitution and polygamy as unsafe sexual habits. The appeal, therefore, is not so much to the old moral polygamous system of the Baganda, but rather to a moral system filled with new rules - but as binding as the old one. Breitinger convincingly draws a parallel between *Give A Chance* and the didactic morality plays of the Middle Ages. This parallel becomes apparent in the two representative figures, Oldpa and Five-Fourteen, who reveal the typical "qualities of the human genus persona" of the morality plays.[52] The form of *Give A Chance* with its questions and answers, also points to its character of a morality play: "This type of question and answer is well known from didactic theory and practice from the 15th century onwards, a didactic technique that has survived in the teaching of the catechism..."[53] Breitinger points out that the AIDS problem has grown to proportions that make it considerably more than just a health issue. It has become a moral issue which is looked upon in the same categories as is done in the biblical plays. In those plays, the sinful life of the people endangers the way to salvation. In Uganda, AIDS

51 Bogatyrev, *The Function of Folk Costume*, p. 95.

52 Breitinger, "Popular Urban Theatre," p. 286.

53 ibid., p. 287; s.a. Mlama, *Culture and Development*.

endangers the physical life of the whole nation. I agree with Breitinger when he concludes it only logical that Ugandan modern morality plays, since they address comparable issues, should also apply "comparable forms of character representation, of plot development in the form of didactic dialoguing, ikonographic labelling of issues."[54]

With the AIDS Quake Festival, APAU's activities did not stop. For the second half of 1990, they planned to conduct workshops in schools.[55] They want to sensitise the pupils to the problem AIDS, to stimulate discussions, and if possible, have the pupils perform short plays themselves. Lennie Kabunga, chairman of APAU, believes it to be considerably more effective to raise consciousness through theatre than by lecturing. The AIDS Quake Festival, which has been recorded on video, and is now edited, is very important in this respect, too, since the video can be used for the campaign in the schools.

4.4.2. *The Riddle*

In April 1991, the School Health Education Project of the Ministry of Education and UNICEF jointly launched a nationwide drama-competition in primary schools. They felt that drama could be an effective way of transmitting information about AIDS to Ugandans through school-children.[56] Contrary to local problems in rural communities, health education projects concern people in the first place as individuals. Poor health conditions and disease become of public interest, however, if they assume epidemic proportions, or if the channels of transmission of the diseases can be located in public institutions - like schools. Target audiences for plays about health education, therefore, have to be defined according to those locations where a high frequency of infections occur.[57] By focussing

---

54 Breitinger, "Popular Urban Theatre," p. 286.

55 The other play performed at the AIDS Quake Festival, *Abajambula mu Lubiri*, was in Luganda. As with *Give A Chance*, it used devices of the morality plays to depict different aspects of AIDS. In this play, the symbol of Kingship is employed to show how AIDS destroys the human body. "The King in his palace is the human body, his soldiers the white blood cells and his enemies the disease. In a typical traditional life style of Kingship, life is full of excesses, love, hate, betrayal and falls prey to a new and invincible enemy, AIDS." The play is suppposed to serve as a warning. s. 1989/1990 Project Report.

56 Sarah K. Birungi, *A Report on AIDS Drama Competition. "The Riddle,"* 1991, unpublished. p. 1.

57 Breitinger, "Popular Urban Theatre," p. 283.

the AIDS Drama competition on primary schools, the organisers tried to address the school-children not only as target audience, but also as multipliers. The objective of the campaign was to warn primary school children of the dangers of AIDS, but also, through the children and through performing and watching the AIDS drama, the parents and communities. An attempt was made to reach all communities with AIDS information, and also to sensitise the Regional and District Officers about the importance of promoting AIDS drama as an instrument of communication. In order to be an incentive for the participation of as many pupils as possible, the organisers designed the campaign in the form of a competition: one play, *The Riddle*, was to be performed by all the primary schools in the country, and the winning groups were given awards.

The competition took place on zonal, county, district, regional and then national level. For the final competition, the winning groups of each region went to the National Theatre in Kampala. The organisers put particular emphasis on the training of the adjudicators who were divided up into three committees. The National AIDS Drama Competition Committee was the main administrative committee, consisting of the National School Health Education Coordinator, two UNICEF members, and six Ugandan drama professionals. This committee briefed regional as well as district adjudicators. In order to train the adjudicators, a two-weeks resident workshop was held at Namagunga Girls School. Participants were supposed to come from all thirty-four districts of Uganda. The workshop intended to train two competent adjudicators from each district to handle organisation, administration and adjudication of the competition at all levels throughout the district.[58] In the workshop, various topics were discussed: marking/adjudication, the role of the adjudicator, the role of theatre,[59] discussion of the script of *The Riddle* and of the music in relation to the script, presentation and interpretation. General education on AIDS was given in films which were shown to the participants. Time was also devoted to the discussion of community involvement. It was agreed that participating schools would perform their productions in their communities after the competition was over. After such shows, there would be time for discussion and comments from the audience.[60] All through the workshop, participants

58 ibid.

59 Birungi reports that there was a general discussion on how theatre can be used to mobilise people by entertaining and educating them at the same time.

60 Birungi, "A Report on AIDS Drama Competition," p. 9.

were divided into small groups and they improvised plays around given themes such as "promiscuity leads to AIDS," "love carefully" etc. The other groups would watch and adjudicate, using the marking scheme which had been drawn up during the workshop.[61]

The designers of the competition thought the play would give the children the necessary information about AIDS, and it was hoped that, by performing it themselves, rather than just watching it, they would internalise the message. The organisers of the AIDS drama project decided to start the campaign in primary schools, because children at this level enjoy drama best since their lives revolve around play. Besides, the organisers were of the opinion that "children at this level also appeal more to parents' emotions, so once they got sensitised through drama, they could easily cause change in their parents' thinking and attitudes."[62]

The title of the play, *The Riddle*, refers to a riddle called *ebikojjo* in Luganda, where children solve a problem through questions and answers.[63] Thus, the title of the play has for children immediate connotations of problem solution. The problem to be solved is, of course, AIDS. One theme of the plot is the competition itself. There are two students, Sezi and Seku, who participate in their school's performance of the play. Sezi's parents suffer from AIDS, and he feels uneasy, whenever the topic AIDS is mentioned. Nevertheless, he frequently has conversations with his friend Seku, where they speak about ways of infection, transmission and prevention of AIDS. More factual knowledge is given by their teacher, Mr. Suubi, during the rehearsals. In one of the classes, he warns the pupils about sugar-daddies/mummies:

> Mr. Suubi: Girls, you need to avoid the older men who are now turning to young girls because they know that the women of their age have already been infected by AIDS. You must learn right now the danger they are likely to get you into... I am emphasizing girls, but boys should be on the look out as well. There are older women who are in to seduce you too...[64]

In several mime scenes, seduction of girls and boys by sugar-daddies/mummies is demonstrated: the sister of one pupil is seduced by a

61 ibid.

62 ibid, p. 2.

63 Mbowa, "Ugandan Literature."

64 Harriet Masembe, *The Riddle. AIDS Drama Competition for Primary Schools 1991* (Kampala: Ministry of Education, School Health Education project, 1991), p. 10.

teacher, Sezi's father is a sugar-daddy and seduces a young girl, and the co-wife of Sezi's mother is a sugar-mummy who seduces a school-boy. Ironically, Mr. Banja, the co-ordinator of the competition, is one of the sugar-daddies the play warns against. He tries to seduce Miss Kazoole, one of the district producers, by promising her undue advantages in the competition. When Miss Kazoole in turn tries to get information from Mr. Suubi about his production by offering him sex, the vicious circle is broken: Mr. Suubi, whose name is the Luganda word for *hope*, refuses. He wants to use the competition for what it is, an instrument to educate and protect the children against AIDS.

In a conversation with Mr. Banja, Miss Kazoole brings up an important issue: whether AIDS can be cured by traditional medicine or not.

> Miss Kazoole: Science has failed, we have to admit that, I am afraid. In the situation we are in, we have no choice but to turn back to our traditional medicine.[65]

Mr Banja contradicts her and stresses that there is no cure for AIDS, and the only chance to conquer the disease lies in making every effort to protect those who are not yet infected.[66]

A key scene of the play is a speech by the Minister of Health to all pupils assembled at Lugogo stadium. By conveying unmistakably all the necessary information about AIDS, the speech is almost an "insert of reality into the fictitious plot":[67]

> Minister: I am made to understand for every 100 Ugandans, 10 are infected with AIDS virus. The age groups most affected are those aged 15 to 40 years who are the breadwinners for their families and indeed this nation. The second most affected group are children below 5 years who are the future pillars of

---

65 ibid., p. 11.

66 Between 1989 and 1991, there were repeated rumours about healers with a cure against AIDS. One of those 'healers,' an old woman called Nanyonga, caused a lot of excitement in November/December 1989. She claimed that she had had a vision of Christ telling her how to cure AIDS-patients with soil. Thousands of AIDS-patients went to see her in the hope to be cured. When she first went public, up to 30000 people had come to her village and camped in front of her hut. Eventually, the Government had to ban Nanyonga's activities. Even the pop-star Philly Lutaaya was accused by journalists of having sought the help of Nanyonga in her village. He declared that this was not true, and in his documentary, Lutaaya stressed that there is no cure against AIDS and that so far the only possible action is to prevent its further spreading. Patrick Mugizi. "Nakivubo cries, laughs, and mocks Lutaaya." *Weekly Topic* (Uganda), November 8, 1989.

67 Breitinger, "Popular Urban Theatre," p. 286.

> this nation. Ladies and Gentlemen, up to this day AIDS has no cure. Fortunately, the modes of transmission are already well known to us as already outlined by the Ministry of Health on many occasions namely:
> a) Sexual contact with an infected person
> b) Infected mother to her newborn baby
> c) Thirdly, through transfusion with contaminated blood and use of unsterilized medical instruments such as needles and syringes...[68]

At the end of the play, Sezi's parents both die of AIDS, and his father's second wife flees to another town: "They say I have caused these deaths. I should go to another town and live there happily before I also die."[69] The script leaves Sezi's future open to be filled in by the respective producers of the play, giving them room for their own ideas and suggestions and challenging them "to come up with an 'imaginative' ending."[70] They are involved in the production in order to overcome the impression that what is expected is merely the performance of a script handed down from above. The open end leaves an opportunity to find a solution that is plausible for the audience in the respective area.

In *The Riddle*, the behaviour of adults is shown as a warning for the school-children. The consequences of promiscuity are demonstrated, for the individual, and more importantly, for others, like partners, and for children who are left behind as orphans.[71] The same is true for polygamous marriages if partners are not faithful.

The strong emphasis on educating the children requires the presentation of themes which are relevant to them - hence the focus on sugar daddies/mummies. Especially in the towns, this phenomenon has become a problem. An increasing number of older men and women seduce school-girls/boys by promising them sweets or money. For these men and women, sex among their own age group looks increasingly dangerous, the seduction of adolescents posing less of a risk. The play tries to warn school-children against those men and women. On a verbal level, the teacher Mr. Suubi explains the danger children face. On the emotional level, they are addressed in the mime scenes where the seduction of young boys and girls

68 *The Riddle*, p. 8.

69 ibid. p. 16.

70 Birungi, "A Report on AIDS Drama Competition," p. 3.

71 Breitinger, "Popular Urban Theatre," p. 286.

by sugar daddies/mummies is enacted visually. In those scenes, both the seduced and the seducers die from AIDS.

The message of the play, to take AIDS information seriously and to live accordingly, is re-enforced by music. Almost all the scenes start with the famous song "Alone" by Philly Lutaaya, where the pop-star advocates openness and information in the fight against AIDS, especially for children, who can still be protected. Besides Philly Lutaaya's song, Uganda now has one song conveying the same message in different languages: the Kazo Nursery Song, in which children appeal to their parents to avoid behaviour that will cause them (the parents) to contract AIDS.[72] The song was composed for the AIDS Drama Competition.

It has to be noted that the concept of the competition did not work as well as expected. Even before the first performances on zonal level began, it became obvious to some participants that the element of competition took priority over the real aim of the play, i.e. AIDS education. The fact that the plays were performed as part of a competition interfered with the actual goal of the project, because the participants tended to act for the adjudicators rather than for the audience. Some up-country schools even did not want to participate at all: they thought that they would not be among the winners. Sarah Birungi accordingly notes that due to the competitive basis, producers and adjudicators paid more attention to the theatre skills than to impact. Besides, it is likely that some good productions were not seen by many people because only one production moved on from every stage to compete at the next level. Even those plays which moved on to the next stages, however, were not seen by big audiences, because they were performed during working hours, so that the adjudicators would have enough time for their work. The two winning productions at the national level, finally, were from Central and Mukono regions.[73] I agree with Briungi when she complains that this was discouraging to the groups from up-country, who may not show their productions again.[74]

Another weakness of the nationwide campaign is the content of the play was not viewed with equal relevance throughout the country. In the city

[72] Birungi, "A Report on AIDS Drama Competition," p. 16; at the National Theatre, the song was sung in eight languages, such as Lugishu, Karimojong, Acholi, Lutoro, Lugbara, Luganda, Lusoga, Runyankole.

[73] The first and second play were shown at the National Theatre in Kampala and at the International Conference Centre to V.I.P.s.

[74] Birungi, "A Report on AIDS Drama Competition," p. 13/14.

of Kampala, for example, sugar daddies/mummies are a well known fact, and the necessity to mention them in a play on AIDS education as a possible source of infection is evident. In an isolated rural area like Karamoja, where we have a different ethnic group and society altogether, sugar daddies/mummies may not be known, and information about them seems irrelevant and incomprehensible, whereas a more common practice in that society may not be addressed.[75]

These shortcomings notwithstanding, it has to be appreciated that all districts of Uganda joined in the competition, and each region was represented at the national level of the competition in Kampala. This means that the message reached many school children, that "at least a big part of the young population in Uganda attending primary school was able to gain some awareness on how AIDS is spread and what can be done in order to control it."[76]

4.5. Plays Addressing a Particular Target-Group

Theatre to support AIDS information is not used in nationwide campaigns only, as the focus on the AIDS Quake Festival and the UNICEF-project in the last chapters might suggest. There are plays written and produced by Ugandans, which address a specific target group. In the following two sub-chapters, examples will be given. It will become clear that they have the same structure and use the same techniques to convey information to the audience. The only distinguishing trait is the characters. In order to arouse the interest of the target group, the characters in the plays belong to these groups - school leavers in the case of Owor's play, and students in Kaganda's play.

4.5.1. *Burdens Of Youth*

Mary F. Owor of the Department of Health Education in the Ministry for Education produced the play *Burdens Of Youth*, by the authors Jackie Wacha and Felicity Okoth, which was shown on Ugandan TV. It addresses those young Ugandans who have just finished school and more often than not are unemployed, despite good exam results. The play begins with some

---

75 Personal interview with Augustine Bazaale, National Theatre, Kampala, 26/8/91.

76 Birungi, "A Report on AIDS Drama Competition," p. 14.

young people trying to find a job. The situation is frustrating: either there are no jobs, or, the available jobs are poorly paid. One of the girls, Susan, tries to escape this situation by letting older men keep her. She eventually becomes infected with AIDS, and the play ends with her friends realizing that Ugandans have to change their sexual behaviour:

Peter:	The most important thing now is to combat the disease. Prevent its spread. We need Health Education now more than ever before. Health Education particularly for the innocent school population and youth who are always victimized.
Betty:	But we also need to help those who are already infected. Educate them so that they don't despair or spread it further.
Peter:	Yes, we are told that AIDS is not spread by mere touching, sharing cups or eating from the same vessels with an infected person. That even kissing does not spread AIDS, unless you have wounds in the mouth.
Betty:	... So all we need to stress is this business of sex which seems to be the major cause. If only we could alter our sex habits...[77]

In *Burdens Of Youth*, two groups are opposed to each other. One, exemplified by Susan, who displays the wrong behaviour allowing older men to keep her in order to escape poverty. The second group is represented by the other school-leavers. They, too, are subjected to poverty, but unlike Susan, they do not resort to prostitution - they still adhere to such principles as 'safe sex' and 'zero grazing.'

Again, the causes of AIDS are seen in promiscuity and the immoral life-style of many Ugandans. As in *The Riddle*, the problem of 'sugar daddies' is addressed. School-leavers are warned, because it is this age-group which is still largely uninfected and in danger of seduction. By opposing the two sets of characters, and showing right moral behaviour as opposed to inappropriate behaviour, the authors convey their message: lead a moral life if you want to live and also stop AIDS. The message, unfortunately, is not as simple as it may appear. The authors acknowledge poverty and unemployment force many women into prostitution, and many men, separated from their families, seek a sexual outlet with prostitutes. Still, they stress that despite these difficult conditions, an effort has to be made to change behaviour and halt the further spreading of the disease. The need for health education is emphasised, especially for the children. As

[77] *Burdens Of Youth*, p. 17.

in *Give A Chance* and *The Riddle,* the importance of changing behavioural practice is conveyed: the play advocates better information for children. It is imperative to alter the prevailing attitude of discouraging children to ask questions. Wacha and Okoth try to influence this attitude by appealing to the traditional value of human continuity: if people want to ensure the principle of human continuity, they have to educate the children about AIDS. The play does not make the usual distinction between immoral promiscuous and moral monogamous behaviour. This can be seen in Betty's statement that it is also necessary to help those already infected. The authors admit the economic and social problems of many people are overwhelming and easily lead to promiscuity, and they stress that in order to survive the AIDS-epidemic, there is no alternative to a changing behaviour. By adopting this attitude, Wacha/Okoth sensibly avoid the contradiction arising by an appeal to morality as a way of making people change their habits. Plays about AIDS have the difficult task of conveying the reason for infection is irresponsible sexual behaviour, while at the same time stressing that victims must not be stigmatized. Obviously, the appeal to morality becomes somewhat ambiguous.

As with the plays already discussed, information in *Burdens Of Youth* is conveyed through dialogue, appealing to the rational part of consciousness. Through conversations among the school-leavers, the medical facts about AIDS are discussed, putting the play in the same category of didactic plays as *Give A Chance*. More than in *Give A Chance* and *The Riddle*, in *Burdens of Youth* the socio-economic causes for the spreading of the disease are acknowledged, thereby placing the suggested solution in a wider context. It is regrettable the play was exclusively shown on TV, where only a small percentage of Ugandans, and of Ugandan school-leavers, could watch it. By limiting the play to the TV medium, the number of spectators was comparatively small, and the advantages inherent in the medium theatre have been sacrificed.[78] As the discussion of the Kamiriithu project showed, not only the content of a message is important.[79] Its effectiveness depends on the medium of communication. By restricting *Burdens Of Youth* to TV, its influence becomes considerably weaker without the personal atmosphere of a live performance, not to speak of participation.

---

78 s. chapter 3.5.

79 s. chapter 2.1.

4.5.2. Kaganda's Play - No Title

Kwezi Kaganda, a 2nd year drama Student at Makerere University in 1990, treats the subject from a similar viewpoint in his play. It is set among students, and, like *Burdens Of Youth*, it begins with a group discussing AIDS. Everybody argues a particular viewpoint: AIDS can be conquered by self-discipline, abstinence, "zero grazing," a religious life-style; one of them does not believe AIDS exists at all; and one of the female students just ignores it. As it turns out, this student is infected, and each of the male students has had sex with her, in spite of his 'personal recipe' against AIDS. The play ends with a warning:

> Mukasa: What has the world gone mad? Yes, the world is mad with worldly pleasure and has forgotten any kind of selfcontrol... About 95% of AIDS is caused by sexual contact. We all know that we should control our sexual behaviour, but knowing what is right is not enough. Doing what is right is the answer and this is only possible through self-discipline. Otherwise you and me can wait for our turns.[80]

What becomes obvious are differences between what people say, and what they actually do - between theory and action. The characters speak of ways to protect themselves. In the end, however, it is revealed that this was only talk while in reality, the lifestyles have not changed. The play exposes patterns of evasion regarding instructions towards a change of behaviour: on a verbal level, people agree, but this does not translate into action. The characters utter the sentences which are expected from people with their level of information and awareness, but this is only outward appearance. In point-of-fact, their behaviour has not changed.

Burdens Of Youth and the play by Kwezi Kaganda have identical structures to bring across information about AIDS. They use the pattern typical for didactic plays, as was seen in *Give A Chance* and *The Riddle*. There are always two types of people in these plays: those who do not know or do not want to know anything about the disease and consequently behave irresponsibly. Then, there is the well-informed person, who is frequently involved with AIDS-education campaigns. From this character comes the factual information appealing to the audience's cognitive system, usually through dialogue with a friend who belongs to the first group. He encourages his friend to change his behaviour, but the friend is not

---

80 Kwezi Kaganda, unpublished play, no title, 1990.

influenced and is eventually infected with the disease. Too late, he regrets his unreasonableness. This is where the affective system of the spectators is addressed. The emotionally involved audience is shocked by his fate, and it is hoped that they draw the obvious conclusion: change their own sexual behaviour or the same will happen to them. That conclusion is presented on stage by others in the group advocating to abandon promiscuity. The solution to the problem of HIV/AIDS can then be tailored to the conditions and circumstances of targeted audiences. By seeing the characters on stage contract AIDS, although infection could have been avoided had they heeded the information given them, the spectators are supposed to draw the necessary conclusions for their own lives. Depending on the target group, the plays are set among different segments of society, e.g. students, workers, pupils etc.

4.6. TFD that Uses Other Media

That *Burdens Of Youth* was shown on TV and not in a theatre hall, points to the fact that increasingly media other than theatre are applied in the fight against AIDS. In the following two chapters, two such projects will be described. I nevertheless decided to place them within the TFD category because they use the same structure and techniques to convey information as the plays previously discussed. What has led them to employ other media, such as film, video and cassettes, is their attempt to disseminate their message more widely.

4.6.1. *It's Not Easy*

Also belonging to the category of plays addressing a particular target group is *It's Not Easy*, produced as a film by the American NGO, *The Experiment in International Living* (EIL). It has been shown on Ugandan TV several times, and EIL teams take it up-country on AIDS-information and mobilisation tours. Other organisations, such as the World Health Organisation, show the video on their AIDS education tours throughout Uganda. WHO uses the opportunity to distribute condoms after the video-show. This usually stimulates discussions among the audience and gives the accompanying health-educators a chance to provide additional information. On some occasions, as many as 5000 to 10 000 people are mobilised.[81]

81 Interview with L.B. Wilson, WHO.

The video-taped play is about two couples who are friends. The husbands are employed in the same office in Kampala, and earn enough money to be able to afford nice bungalows in the suburbs. One of the wives, Serra, is pregnant, the other couple already has a daughter. They meet frequently in the evenings to talk or play cards. One evening, they have a discussion about AIDS. One of the men, Suna, tries to play down the problem and even refuses to listen to information about the disease. He is certain he is not infected, because he feels healthy. The other husband, Magezi, is engaged in AIDS education, and tries to explain that feeling healthy does not necessarily mean that one is not infected since it may take a long time for AIDS symptoms to appear. After that evening, Suna and Magezi have many conversations about AIDS in which Magezi wants to make his friend aware of the danger in which he places himself and others through his attitude. Magezi knows that Suna has many girl-friends, and throughout the film, there are conversations, when Magezi tries to persuade Suna to change his behaviour. As in the plays discussed before, factual information about AIDS is conveyed through dialogue.

Shortly after Serra has given birth, doctors discover that both she and the baby have AIDS, and that it was Suna who infected them. He then realises the results of his irresponsibility: he is the cause for both his wife's and the baby's eventual death, but the insight comes too late.

The second half of the film deals with the problem of how to behave towards infected people. Again, information is conveyed to the audience through dialogue between the characters. Magezi convinces Suna that he has to inform his colleagues and his boss about his infection. After the revelation, some of Suna's colleagues refuse to have contact with him because they fear they might become infected. They do not pay attention to Magezi who explains that the only modes of transmission are through blood and sex. The boss is more understanding. When he learns of Suna's infection he uses it as an opportunity to call a meeting of company directors, in order to discuss what is to be done with HIV-positive members of staff. In the end, they decide to support Suna, since the disease is not spread by using the same toilet facilities, eating the same food, etc., and the other workers are therefore not endangered.

In order to raise consciousness among the spectators, in *It's Not Easy* the same combination of appeals both to cognitive as well as affective systems are made. The play provides factual information about the disease, but the emotional impact is through the audience's identification with Suna's wife and baby. Serra, a pretty housewife who has no influence on the behaviour of her husband, now has to suffer for his actions. The real victim, however, is the baby. Once again, the empathy of the audience is stirred by an appeal made to traditional moral values.

It's Not Easy differs from the other plays discussed in this chapter in two respects mainly. First, the play was not produced as a theatre play, but as a screen play, which can be shown as video and on TV. The producers, in their attempt to spread AIDS information as widely as possible, thought that by doing so, the message would reach far more people all over the country, than by merely performing it in theatre halls. Since the video has been given to other organisations like WHO and Ugandan TV (UTV), even more people will be exposed to the message. When the video is shown by NGOs in the villages, health educators are present so that a post-performance discussion can take place even though there is no actual life-performance. The production of *It's Not Easy* as a screen-play serves several purposes. Since it's transmission is not limited to TV, the advantages of a live performance could be retained, and there are still discussions after the show. In fact, more people can thus be reached, because it is comparatively cheap to show the play in many communities. The presence of health educators for the discussions is sufficient, no acting-groups have to be taken up-country. Besides, the entertainment value of a video is probably bigger than that of a theatre performance. A video is associated with progress and modernity by a village audience - it is a substitute for the cinemas of the big cities. Another attraction is that in a screen play it is possible to use more sophisticated props than on a simple village-stage. The setting thus offers more visual stimulants. With *It's Not Easy*, EIL managed to exploit the advantages of the medium theatre, while at the same time improving on them.

The other difference to the plays discussed earlier is the strong focus on the negative treatment and behaviour towards people infected with AIDS. In *It's Not Easy*, it is still stressed that the main cause for the spread of the disease is promiscuity. As in *Burdens Of Youth*, however, there is not a very strong emphasis on morality, rather the social implications of the high number of AIDS-infections in Uganda are exposed. It is clear that with the high number of infections, there is no room for prejudice. For example, there are long scenes where Suna's colleagues avoid him when they learn of his infection, and Magezi tries to educate them about the channels of transmission. He, and later the boss at the meeting of directors, reiterate that it is safe to live and work together with HIV-positive people since AIDS is only transmitted through sex:

Boss:	... We can no longer afford to sack employees who are found to be infected with the AIDS virus. Not only is it unethical, but also it does not make good business sense. The cost of training new personnel to replace those who are sacked is very expensive. The fact is, a person infected with the AIDS virus is capable of providing valuable service to the company for many years. Those infected are of no risk to fellow workers, providing everyone is made aware of the facts of how the virus is transmitted. We need AIDS education, training, counselling for those infected or feeling at risk, and above all we need commitment at the management level...[82]

At home, Suna's wife is exposed to the same prejudices: her friend, Vicky, at first avoids seeing her and does not want her little daughter to visit her anymore for fear of infection. Eventually, after discussions with her husband, Magezi, where the ways of transmission are again stated, she realises her behaviour is wrong:

Vicky:	They're sick Magezi. My God, they have AIDS. What if we already got it from them?
Magezi:	Vicky. You know we can't catch AIDS from socializing with Suna and Serra.
Vicky:	But, what about Amy? Suna always hugs and kisses her.
Magezi:	It's perfectly safe. The only way we could catch it is if we were exposed to their blood, or through sexual contact. You know that.
Vicky:	I'm just not comfortable...
Magezi:	You remember what the counsellor told us. The virus can pass between people during sexual contact. This is the most common way it is spreading. Another way is if you get infected blood into your blood-stream; like through a blood transfusion if the blood has not been tested, or if you have an injection with an unsterilized needle, or likewise when a traditional healer uses an unsterilized blade.[83]

The target-audience of *It's Not Easy* seems to be the new middle-class that emerged in post-Civil War Uganda. That middle-class comprises such professional groups as accountants, small businessmen, office-clerks working

82 John Riber. *It's Not Easy*, unpublished script, 1991. p. 39.

83 ibid., p. 32/33.

for international organisations or NGOs and therefore having good salaries. The characters in the film belong to that middle-class as can clearly be seen in the setting and the dress they wear: they live in pretty bungalows in the suburbs, a privilege not many Ugandans have, and they wear urban/Western dress. The film does not try to enhance a feeling of national identity in the audience by presenting some of the attributes of Ganda-culture, like traditional dress.

While *It's Not Easy* may work very well with city-audiences, the question has to be asked if it is equally relevant for spectators in the rural areas. The film apparently serves the purpose of leading to discussions between audience and health educators on information tours up-country. It appears to me, however, that those information campaigns could be even more effective if a film more oriented towards the target groups in the villages were shown.

4.6.2. Philly Lutaaya

Philly Lutaaya, the noted Ugandan pop-star, went a step further in his use of media. He stressed that information is the most powerful weapon in the fight against AIDS. Between late 1989 and the early months of 1990, his song "Alone" could be heard all over Kampala - in markets, taxis, shops, bars, and on buses. Having learned he was suffering from AIDS he initiated an extensive AIDS-information campaign, using himself as a warning example. A series of concerts followed the release of the cassette, with the profits going into AIDS-research and information. *Alone* was produced with the financial help of the Swedish Red Cross and part of its profits went to the Ugandan Red Cross and the Ministry of Health's AIDS Control Programme to sponsor further AIDS information campaigns. In the titlesong of the cassette, "Alone," Philly argues for information:

Chorus:

Today it's me, tomorrow someone else
It's me and you, we got to stand out and fight
We'll shed a light in the fight against AIDS
Let's come on out, let's stand together and fight AIDS
In times of joy, in times of sorrow
let's take a stand and fight on to the end
With open hearts let us stand out
And speak out to the world - we'll save some lives
Save the children of the world

Let's be open, advise the young ones
A new generation to protect and love
Hear them singing, playing, laughing
Let's give them everything in truth and love.

As with the plays, Philly's song stresses the importance of protecting children by being open and educating them about AIDS which can only be conquered by a joint effort: "Let's stand together," he says and appeals to traditional Ganda values, such as human solidarity and the responsibility to ensure the survival of society through the children. Solidarity is necessary to create a better future. In a country with high illiteracy, music is a good media to spread a message. The tune of "Alone" is easy to remember so everybody can join in when the song is played. It's structure follows that of traditional Bantu songs with its change between one singer and the chorus where everybody can participate. In order to reach more people with the message, "Alone" was translated into Luganda, the lingua franca in the south and southwest of Uganda.

Another part of the AIDS information campaign was the production of a film about Philly Lutaaya's life which describes how he returned to Uganda after the civil war from his exile in Sweden. The fact he returned, and it was again possible to attend open-air concerts without risking one's life, made Lutaaya a symbol of peace to many Ugandans. Aware of the rapid spread of AIDS and its taboo nature in Uganda, he decided to come out and declare publicly that he was suffering from it. In 1988 even more than today, AIDS was associated with immorality and those infected tried not to let anybody know about it.[84] Philly Lutaaya hoped his openness could contribute to the prevention of further infections by demonstrating that indeed anyone can be infected with AIDS. He was supported and encouraged in his campaign by the World Health Organisation and the International Red Cross. The film shows problems he faced after his declaration on April 13th 1989; people simply did not believe him, and the press thought his declaration was a public-relations-trick. Those who did believe him, like Ms. Amana of the World Health Organisation/Global Programme on AIDS, encouraged him to go on with his campaign. During this time, he gave numerous speeches, directed primarily to school-children and students; in a speech at Makerere University he addressed 5000 students. Eventually, his message took root and people began to believe

84 Noreen Kaleeba, founder of TASO, in the documentary. TASO is a Ugandan self-help group for AIDS victims that has gained world-wide recognition.

him. When he decided to make a film to further spread his message, he was confronted with another problem: the Ugandan Government opposed the idea for fear that Uganda might appear to be the AIDS-capital of the world. After negotiations and correspondence with the Prime Minister, it was realised that only an open policy towards AIDS could prevent its further spreading, and Government supported the documentary, the Prime Minister being present at its first screening and President Museveni becoming the first African president to openly acknowledge the problem AIDS.

For Philly Lutaaya, the production of the film and the cassette, was a way to express his feeling of helplessness and loneliness; it was also a way to inform Ugandans of the disease. The film contains footage of Lutaaya in concert, during public talks addressing students, school-children, villagers, and sometimes speaking directly to the camera. This is supplemented by footage of other people's comments on Philly Lutaaya and on AIDS. There are, e.g., interviews with Ms. Amana from WHO/GPA, speaking about her organisation's involvement in the campaign, and with Noreen Kaleeba, founder of TASO.

In the documentary Lutaaya again emphasises that information and education about the disease are crucial to control and prevent its spread. Although he admits sexual behaviour of Ugandans during the last years has been too free, thereby giving AIDS a chance to spread, he opposes a moral judgement of AIDS-victims. He points out that blame is not productive: directing energy and resources to the fight against AIDS is more worthwhile. The producers of the documentary try to encourage a feeling of solidarity in Ugandans by talking at length about the attitude of the Ugandan Government towards the documentary. The fact that the Government at first opposed it, is discussed openly, but it is made clear now the Ugandan Government under President Museveni has adopted an exceptionally open policy in the fight against AIDS - unequalled by any other African country and most western countries. Uganda does outstanding things in the fight against AIDS.[85] It is a challenge to Ugandans to live up to those high standards and to conquer the disease by a change of personal

85 Due to the open attitude towards AIDS, information and education campaigns could be carried out so that a high standard of information was achieved. Another accomplishment is the screening of the Nakasero Blood Bank, which makes blood-transfusions safe again. Besides, the self-help group TASO was founded, which by now is so renowned that many foreign journalists come to Uganda to report about its work.

behaviour. The feeling of pride in the country which Philly tries to create could form the basis for a greater attitude of solidarity.

Only a few public figures all over the world have declared they have AIDS, Philly was the first prominent African to admit he was infected. He lived in real life what the characters in the plays discuss. He used his own experience as a warning to save the lives of those not yet infected. With his declaration and campaign, he not only appealed to the Ganda value of solidarity, he embodied it. To spread his message, Philly used all media available to him: music, cassettes (audio and video), film, lectures. Today he is known not only throughout Uganda, but in other parts of the world too for his courageous campaign. His songs were on the minds of everybody in Uganda, and that a person of such stature could be infected with AIDS made it clear that nobody was safe from the disease. The impact of Lutaaya's declaration becomes clear when compared to the stir caused by the 'coming out' of the American basketball star, Magic Johnson. Like Philly, Magic Johnson is an idol and a symbol of success. Philly used his popularity as an instrument to demonstrate publicly the values to be adopted in order to save society: he has become a symbol in the fight against AIDS by giving "the disease a public face."[86] Philly Lutaaya died on December 15th 1989.

Lutaaya's campaign did not include theatre in its pure form. I have nevertheless discussed it, because, in my opinion, it gives an outlook on the future development of Campaign Theatre. Philly Lutaaya has carried the two basic characteristics of CT to their most extreme point: first, he succeeded in reaching numerous audiences with his message by travelling through the country and speaking with as many people as possible. Moreover, the documentary was shown on TV, and NGOs and international organisations like WHO continue showing the video on information tours, so a large part of the Ugandan population has now seen it; and secondly, Lutaaya developed the characteristic of TFD to go beyond the purely theatrical event, further by employing media other than theatre. The aim of Campaign Theatre to reach many people as well as the technological progress which allows for the integration of video, film, cassettes etc., suggests that Philly Lutaaya's campaign set the tone for the future.

---

86 Noreen Kaleeba in the documentary.

4.7. Plays for Conscientisation - Plays about AIDS

4.7.1. Summary of the Case Studies

The case studies show that to raise consciousness, the same structures, techniques and plots are applied in each of the plays discussed. With the exception of Philly Lutaaya's film, all the plays have two sets of characters opposed to each other: there are those characters who are informed about AIDS and know they have to behave responsibly in order to stop the disease, and in contrast, there is the character, who does not recognise the threat of AIDS and who, through his or her sexual behaviour, is infected and endangers the life of those who are in sexual contact with him/her. By contrasting these attitudes, information about protecting oneself and others is given. The information conveyed in those discussions clearly appeals to the cognitive, rational part of the spectators' consciousness. By educating the audience through dialogue, song, dance and mime, the plays continue using devices common in educative drama since the Middle Ages. The spectators are not left in doubt about which view-point to adopt. If not earlier, then at last when one of the characters gets infected with the disease as a result of his/her personal behaviour, they are made to realise the character who is well-informed and careful in his/her sexual habits reflects the proper attitude. This device is taken to its most extreme by Philly Lutaaya who used his own situation as a warning. The information is repeated several times, not only on the verbal level, but also in songs, dances and mime-scenes thereby working on all the senses. By keeping the language simple, the authors presume that the message comes across to everybody in the audience. This is also reflected in the type of English used, i.e. the Ugandan version of English, not standard English. The message is conveyed through Ugandan metaphors and proverbs as well as references to persons well-known to a Ugandan audience. In nearly all current plays, e.g. Philly Lutaaya is either mentioned or his song "Alone" is played.

As seen with the AIDS Quake Festival which was recorded on video, theatre artists involved in AIDS education rely increasingly on media other than theatre. The trend continues with the film *It's Not Easy* by EIL, and also in Philly's campaign. These examples show the direction which CT will take in the future: in order to reach larger audiences with their message, artists employ a combination of different media. The importance of these campaigns is obvious in a country like Uganda, where a large proportion of the population is illiterate and only a small percentage of the people has access to TV and radio.

All the plays stress AIDS is transmitted through sexual intercourse. As a solution, they suggest a monogamous life-style to prevent the further spread of the disease. All are based on the recognition that Ugandans lead a promiscuous life-style and must be conscientised to change behaviour and adhere to principles like "zero grazing" and "love carefully." On the cognitive level, the playwrights try to convince spectators they have to change by giving them essential facts about the transmission of AIDS. On the affective, subconscious level, the appeal is to traditional moral values of Ganda-society, i.e. the principle of human continuity, solidarity and social responsibility. The strong focus on educating children, especially those of school-age serves that purpose. Accordingly, children are a target-group of particular importance. All plays stress the children are as yet HIV/AIDS-free and can still be protected from the disease. The necessity to lay special emphasis on the education of school-children before they become sexually active is obvious, but the fact that only about forty per cent of all children in Uganda attend school must also be considered. Consequently, the concentration of information campaigns on schools only is not effective, as it is equally important to reach those children who never go to school. That was attempted in the WHO-APAU project. The AIDS Quake Festival addressed its message to all age-groups.[87] There was to be a follow-up, however, to educate children: the edited video of the festival is to be shown in schools, but street-children and market boys are also planned to be involved.[88]

Since there is no cure for AIDS, as a solution the plays emphasise the further spreading of the disease has to be stopped; this can only be achieved by a change of sexual behaviour. The plays all argue that Ugandans during the years of turmoil, diverted from correct moral behaviour and now must return to it.

---

87 Due to the large number of participants belonging to different social and age-groups, and also to the general entertainment character, the festival was not target-specific.

88 Market boys are young boys, usually between 10 and 16 years who work in Nakasero Market in Kampala. Nakasero is one of Kampala's biggest and most expensive markets where mostly ex-patriates go shopping. The market boys wait in the parking-area for the customers and help them carrying their shopping bags, thus earning some money to pay their school-fees or contribute to the family-income.

4.7.2. Evaluation of the Case Studies

In Uganda it is realised that an open attitude, information and education are requisite in the fight against AIDS. This begs the question why, in spite of the numerous information-campaigns, the disease continues to increase.

One reason for the apparently unsatisfactory success of the campaigns is that they are too focussed on Kampala. Projects are usually designed in Kampala, and frequently the authors have the conditions of Kampala in mind when creating the plays. The projects may therefore be adequate for people in the urban centres, but not for those in the rural areas. Many TFD-projects remain in Kampala rather than travelling all over the country. The UNICEF-project, in its attempt to involve all primary schools in the country, seems to have been effective, although its message may not be equally relevant all over Uganda.[89] The same applies to *It's Not Easy*. Philly Lutaaya's documentary shown on information tours in rural areas represents a successful attempt to reach more people.

Writing about a World Vision project on AIDS awareness through drama, the reporter Mkanju mentions the "inhouse trend" of these projects.[90] By using that term to characterize CT, he points to one of its major problems, namely, that, due to the involvement of international organisations and NGOs, many projects do not go beyond festivals like for instance the AIDS Quake. Those festivals are a way to measure success for the organisers which can be reported to headquarters. Mkanju deplores the fact that many "theatre to the people" campaigns have not reached the people, and concludes that there cannot be any meaningful result so long as this trend is not reversed. Obviously, the "inhouse trend" of CT is a problem inherent in that kind of theatre. Since it is connected to NGOs and other international organisations, who bring with them their own organisational pressures, it entails a preference for extravaganzas and a centralised organisation of the campaigns rather than many decentralised small projects. The scholar Kees Epskamp accordingly regards this centralization of the messages as one of the basic contradictions of CT: on the one hand, the messages are conveyed to the audiences on a national level in festivals, drama competitions etc. On the other hand, goals like health care, family planning or the prevention of STDs are not realised nationally but locally,

---

89 s. chapter 4.4.2.

90 Mkanju's report about the second annual AIDS Drama Festival in August at the Concert Hall of the Kenya National Theatre, in *The Sunday Nation*, August 25, 1991.

since they are closely connected to a change of individual behaviour and decisions.[91] For that reason, direct interaction between communicators and audience is essential. Only if the communicator has instant feed-back from the audience he can convey the message according to the mood of the spectators. In this Epskamp sees the reason for the failure of many centralised campaigns where the information is dictated from above. In my opinion, this needs to be seen more differentiated. I agree with Epskamp as far as the big festivals and TV shows are concerned. The case is different, however, if a play like *It's Not Easy, Give A Chance,* or Philly Lutaaya's documentary are shown by NGOs on their up-country information tours. On those occasions, attempts are made to overcome the "inhouse trend," since health-educators are present to discuss the information given in the play with the spectators. It is possible to make adjustments to the reaction of the audience. This device however also points to the weakness of centralised campaigns: they have to be modified when shown to different audiences to be effective. CT by definition is opposed to development and communication projects on a local level: "Whereas in the national campaigns theatre was made for the population, in development projects with a target-group policy there was a preference for theatre made with or by the local population."[92]

Mkanju draws attention to the fact that with a topic as sensitive as AIDS, what is said to a target audience has to be scrutinised carefully so as to avoid misinterpretation or negative information. There may be misconceptions and misunderstandings, especially with nationwide projects like *The Riddle*. Sometimes it happens, especially in comedies, that in references to AIDS women are blamed for the disease. Wrong messages like that could be avoided by sensitizing artists through workshops, as it was done in the WHO-APAU project and in the AIDS Drama Competition. There, the artists openly discussed mistaken information and were given accurate facts. The risk of misconceptions cannot be eliminated completely, because once the workshops for artists and health-educators are over, they work independently. If for example, health-educators in the country, who for religious reasons oppose the idea of birth control, do not pass along the information that condoms are a protection against AIDS, nothing can be done to reverse the influence of those educators.

91 Epskamp, *Theatre in Search for Social Change*,p. 163.

92 ibid., p. 170.

Another reason for the apparent ineffectiveness of the campaigns is that they are too narrowly focussed. They emphasise that promiscuity as the cause for transmission has to stop, that people have to go back to a moral life-style and be monogamous. The complicated nature of this argument has been discussed. The most extreme case is JK Ebonita's video-clip where the messages given on the cognitive and affective level contradict each other: a return to the once functioning traditional value-system is suggested, but with images belonging to city-life and Western culture.[93]

An attempt to include a wider context is made in *Burdens Of Youth* where the authors acknowledge socio-economic problems are involved in the fast spread of AIDS. I believe this part of the problem should be mentioned and discussed more extensively in plays if they are to be relevant to the audience. It is not sufficient for a play to merely give facts about the transmission of AIDS and propose a monogamous life-style as solution. To give spectators the impression their problems are acknowledged and addressed, the social and economic contexts must be included in the plots, as was done in *Burdens Of Youth*. The plays then have stronger relevance to reality. Now, they remain superficial, educating about symptoms rather than causes. Information is given on condom use, treatment of infected people, ways of transmission, and about the necessity to change sexual behaviour to prevent the further spread. As Awam Amkpa has pointed out, AIDS is treated as a cause rather than as a consequence of social and political mishaps.[94] In investigating the high number of AIDS victims in some African countries, one realises that a reason it spreads so quickly is poverty. Many people in Africa cannot afford a balanced diet, and their general physical condition is weaker than that of people in industrialised countries. Resistance, not only against AIDS, but also malaria, diarrhoea is low - also due to the low standard of sanitation and public health. Moreover, medical treatment, when available, is frequently inadequate and unaffordable. One consequence of which is a high prevalence of sexually transmitted diseases, another reason for the rapid spread of AIDS.

When discussing AIDS and the effectiveness of theatre against AIDS in Uganda, the political situation of the last two decades has to be taken into account. Political unrest and civil war led to the decline of social and moral values. As a consequence, Uganda has a large army which, particularly

---

93 s. chapter 4.3.

94 Awam Amkpa, conference at Bayreuth, 13/7/91.

before 1986, was undisciplined - looting, robbing, raping, thereby contributing to the rapid spread of AIDS. Many of the commanders of the National Resistence Army have already died of the disease.

Other social factors are also not being addressed in the plays. One is that Uganda, due to its geographical location, is a country with a high motor freight transit-rate; the highway leading from the coast in Kenya to Zaire, Rwanda, and Central Africa passes through Uganda. In villages where lorry drivers stop for food and rest, there is a high incidence of promiscuity and AIDS. It seems to me that for the campaign propagating a change of sexual behaviour in Uganda to be effective, groups like soldiers, lorry drivers etc. have to be targeted.[95] Although it is most important to educate the children, the further spread of AIDS can only be stopped when society changes its collective sexual behaviour.

Another aspect to be addressed more fully in the plays is the treatment and attitude towards those people who already are infected. The approach adopted in *It's Not Easy* and in Philly Lutaaya's campaign is prudent. Both stress HIV-positive people must not be stigmatised and must remain integrated into society. In *It's Not Easy*, this is unmistakably emphasised in the meeting of directors, when they decide not to dismiss employees infected with AIDS. The strong focus on the behaviour towards those people already suffering from AIDS makes sense when keeping in mind that between 17% and 23% of Ugandans are HIV-positive. In some districts, e.g. Rakai in the south-west, are villages with only children and old people. The old people are too weak to look after the fields, with the result that large agricultural areas are dormant. As AIDS continues to spread, the same is to be expected to happen in other districts.[96] Under these circumstances, rather than stigmatizing AIDS-victims a way of living with them has to be found.[97] Support and understanding are necessary now - a message that needs to be stressed in the plays.

---

95 To my knowledge, this was not done between 1989 and early 1991 when I carried out my research. I am informed, however, that WHO/GPA et al. have refocussed with special emphasis on the following groups: children, taxi and lorry drivers, soldiers, policemen etc.

96 s. "Das Land der leeren Dörfer. Aidstod in Uganda," report by Stefan Spruck, *Weltjournal* Nr. 22 - 4/12/91, shown on German TV (NDR).

97 In some of the villages in Rakai, people who suffer from AIDS are excluded form the village community; they live outside the villages and only get food from the people in the village; s.a. Stefan Spruck, p. 4.

Despite some criticism of TFD on AIDS information, I do not wish to imply that information campaigns are not important; as many people as possible must be educated so they can protect themselves and help those who are already infected. On this point, I do not agree with Mkanju when he warns the AIDS campaign not to become one of the "noises" of our time: "People who live by railway lines and near airports cease to hear their noise." As there is no vaccine against AIDS, people must be taught how to avoid infection. TFD can be an effective instrument serving that purpose, especially when it is not restricted to the purely theatrical level, but can use other media. The projects discussed, should not be considered as seven individual projects, but as a combined, allbeit uncoordinated, effort in the fight against AIDS. Viewed as a whole, with their different approaches and use of various media, their message will reach more and more people all over Uganda.

5. Conclusion

In his address to the United Nations General Assembly, Makagiansar argues for the integration of cultural values into educational processes.[1] He stressed strategies must be found which "make possible the full incorporation of the values of the rural, working, urban and suburban sectors, of the messages of contemporary creation, and of the means of expression of daily life within the formal and non-formal educational processes." Furthermore, the report acknowledges the importance of communication in the modern world, and its interplay with the development of cultural values. Makagiansar points out that in several regional conferences of Unesco, the links between communication and culture have been brought out, and that there can be no cultural policies without communication policies.[2]

In my opinion, the rise of TFD during the last decade has to be understood within that context. As opposed to large-scale development projects, TFD takes the socio-cultural background of the target communities into account, thereby acknowledging the existence of cultural diversity and a plurality of cultures. It represents an integrated approach to both development and communication by being either performed by members of the target community, or as is the case with CT, at least have direct interaction with the audience in post-performance discussions. The advantages of using folk-media, like theatre, for communication in development processes are evident: they are part of the life-style and the culture of the people; their low cost makes it possible to apply them regularly; and because of direct interaction between communicator and audience they have a high potential of persuasiveness.[3]

In the course of this work, I have described the emergence of Campaign Theatre, as a sub-genre of Theatre for Development, in the specific Ugandan context. The survey of theatre in Uganda from 1968 to 1991 was intended to demonstrate the political, social, and cultural forces at work that have led to the phenomenon of CT. As a result of the twenty years of civil war, there is no continuous development in Ugandan theatre.

---

1 Makaminian Makagiansar, reading the report of the Director General of Unesco, in *Cultures*, Vol. VI (Paris: The Unesco Press and la Baconnière, 1979).

2 ibid., p. 15.

3 Kees Epskamp, *Theatre in Search of Social Change*, p. 162.

The influence of the literary dramatists of the sixties and seventies on present-day theatre productions is prevalent, nevertheless. Playwrights, actors and audience alike are familiar with *The Song of Wankoko* or Fajil Mandy's plays, which even today are regularly performed. Other plays, such as those by Robert Serumaga and Nuwa Sentongo, are still remembered by the older generation, and many of the younger playwrights know at least the playscripts through their study of Music, Dance and Drama at Makerere University. The literary dramatists, therefore, had an impact on TFD today - allbeit not discernible at first sight. The difference that strikes one in an initial superficial comparison, can be explained by the different political situations. The playwrights who worked under the oppressive regimes of Obote and Amin wanted to disguise political comment by their use of dramatic techniques, whereas theatre artists today employ strategies with the aim to communicate more clearly to their audience. It is for this reason today's playwrights adapted and developed, rather than merely imitated methods first used by the older playwrights - especially those playwrights' dynamic approach to folklore. This adaptation of theatrical methods ensures that modern productions fit into today's political and social framework. The survey in the first chapter intended to show the political and social conditions in Uganda during the last twenty years that have led to the emergence of present-day Campaign Theatre, with its characteristic organizational and theatrical structures.

After having described CT about AIDS both from theoretical and practical viewpoints, I will summarise some of its basic characteristics. A look at the case studies shows that in Uganda two ways of dealing with the topic AIDS through theatre can be discerned. One is exemplified by the productions of commercial popular theatre groups, like JK Ebonita, the other by the plays produced in cooperation with international organizations and NGOs, i.e. *Give a Chance*, *The Riddle*, et al. I have made it clear that, in my opinion, only the second group falls under the category Theatre for Development/Campaign Theatre. This distinction, however, poses the question of what actually defines a TFD play as opposed to other plays presenting the same topic.

One important difference is the kind of appeal made to the audience. TFD plays apply structures, techniques and plots in order to involve the audience both on an emotional and cognitive level. Through identification with the characters on stage, the spectators are hoped to draw the intended conclusions for their own lives. A play like *The Dollar*, on the other hand, appeals to the audience on another level. It depicts social settings that are decidedly above the aspirations of most Ugandans. The audience follows the action with interest, tension and amusement, but it does not see its own life depicted in the play. This emotional distance, combined with the comical way in which the topic AIDS is presented in *The Dollar*, has the effect that the audience laughs off the problem, rather than being motivated for discussions, not to speak of a change of behaviour.

Another difference is that a TFD play, in order to fulfill its aim to raise consciousness and eventually achieve a change of behaviour in the target audience, focusses exclusively on one topic - AIDS in our case. Its structural presentation follows that of development projects. It is presented to the audience in simple, unmistakable language, e.g. what the problem is, how it came into existence, what can be done to prevent or to solve it. Plays like *The Dollar* or *The Wedshock* do not have this straight-forward structure; they comprise a number of quite unrelated episodes addressing a wide range of topics. The problem AIDS in these plays, is merely displayed and made the subject of a joke. No information that would encourage a change of behaviour is passed along to the audience. The case is slightly different with Ebonita's video-clip which was produced for World AIDS Day. In the video, information about cause and prevention of AIDS is given, and the spectators are admonished to change their behaviour. Nevertheless, there is a difference between the video and TFD plays, as far as production techniques are concerned. Ebonita uses expensive and complicated stage technology as well as elaborate costumes to increase the entertainment value of the show and attract larger audiences. In TFD - both in project-oriented as well as in CT - the productions are far simpler. Especially in CT, where money is spent for the managerial framework and the organisation of the project, so that a play can be performed as often as possible, in many places, always conveying the same message. This desire to expose large audiences to an always identical message, resembles that of commercials. It is, in fact, one of the more important aspects of CT, which was particularly evident in the AIDS Drama Competition *The Riddle*. A play was designed to educate about origins and prevention of AIDS, and by giving the text to all the primary schools to perform, it was ensured that exactly the same message reached increasingly large audiences all over Uganda.

In conclusion, I would like to point-out that Theatre for Development and its sub-genre Campaign Theatre cannot be regarded as idependent of current development politics. To stress this relationship, however, does not mean to minimise the actual achievements of theatre nor its potential. Through theatre, changes are brought about more easily than through lectures, radio, newspapers.[4] Theatre involves people, and motivates them to action - which is, afterall, its objective.

4 ibid., p. 170.

Bibliography

Primary Sources

Bamwesigye, Jones M.R. *The Wish*. unpublished.

Born in Africa. Documentary about Philly Lutaaya (Video).

Bukenya, Austin. *The Bride*. Nairobi: East African Publishing House, 1984.

Ebonita. Videos of musicshows and *The Dollar*.

Kaganda, Kwezi. unpublished play, no title, 1990.

Kasule, Sam. *The Well*. Unpublished, 1989.

Kateete, David. *Give A Chance*. Unpublished play, 1989. Video and script.

Kawadwa, Byron. *St. Lwanga*. Unpublished, 1969.

Kawadwa, Byron and Wessanyi Serukenya. *The Song of Wankoko*. Kampala: The Ministry of Culture and Community Development, 1977.

Kyeyune, Eli N. *Kintu. Legend of the Nile*. Unpublished.

Lutaaya, Philly. *Alone*. Audio-cassette, 1989.

Lwanga-Kizza, Eria. *Women Liberator*. Unpublished, 1985.

Mandy, M. Fagil. *Endless Night*. Unpublished, 1980.

Mandy, Fagil. *Bush Trap*. Unpublished, 1989.

Masembe, Harriet. *The Riddle. AIDS Drama Competition for Uganda Primary Schools 1991*. Kampala: Ministry of Education, School Health Education Project, 1991.

P'Bitek, Okot. *The Horn of My Love*. London: Heinemann (AWS 147); Exeter, NH: Heinemann Inc., 1974.

P'Chong, Cliff Lubwa. *The Bishop's Daughter*. Unpublished.

Riber, John. *It's Not Easy*. Unpublished script, 1991. Video.

Ruganda, John. *The Burdens*. Nairobi, Oxford, New York: Oxford University Press, 1972.

Ruganda, John. *Black Mamba*. *Covenant with Death*. Nairobi: East African Publishing House, 1973.

Ruganda, John. *Echoes of Silence*. Nairobi: Heinemann, 1986.

Ruganda, John. *The Floods*. Nairobi: Heinemann Kenya, 1988.

Sentongo, Nuwa. *The Invisible Bond*. In *African Plays for Playing 1: Hevi, Ajibade, Sentongo*. Ed. Michael Etherton. London: Heinemann, 1975. pp. 8-44.

Serumaga, Robert. *Majangwa and A Play*. Nairobi: East African Publishing House, 1974.

Soyinka, Wole. *A Play of Giants*. London, New York: Methuen, 1984.

Wacha, Jackie and Felicity Okoth. *Burdens Of Youth*. Unpublished.

Zirimu, Elvania Namukwaya. *Family Spear*. Unpublished.

Zirimu, Elvania Namukwaya. *The Poultry Farmer*. Unpublished.

Secondary Sources

A Report on APAU Workshop. 25th - 27th September, 1989. IEC - ACP.

Abah, S. Oga. "Popular Theatre as Integration and Conscientation: The Example of the Katsina-Ala (Nigeria) Project." *Ifda dossier*, 43, July/August 1985. pp. 3-14.

Ahmadu Bello Collective. "Plays for Farmers: Popular Drama Workshops in Northern Nigeria. Stage One: the Ahmadu Bello Initiative." *Théâtre International*, no. 6, 2, 1982. pp. 21-24.

Albrecht, Milton C., James H. Barnett, Mason Griff (eds.). *The Sociology of Art and Literature*. London: Duckworth, 1970 (second impression 1982).

Alphonso, G. "The Training of Barefoot Doctors." *Adult Education and Development*, 1979, no. 12. pp. 43-45.

Awa, N.E. "Bringing Indigenous Knowledge into Planning." *Media Development*, 1, 1987. pp. 22-24.

Baker, S. "Belly Laughs on an Empty Stomach." *Guardian: Third World Review*, 21, May 1979.

Bame, K.N. "Comic Plays in Ghana: an Indigenous Art Form for Rural Social Change." *Rural Africana*, 27, 1975. pp. 25-41.

Banham, Martin. *African Theatre Today*. London: Pitman Publishing, 1976.

Barber, Karin. "Popular Arts in Africa." *African Studies Review*, Vol. 30, no. 3, September 1987. pp. 1-78.

Bazaale, Augustine. "Ugandan Theatre - Structure and Organisation." paper presented to The Conference of Theatre Data, 6-8 July 1988.

Belal, Abdul Aziz. "Culture and Development: an Approach to Under-Development." In *Cultures* Vol. VI, no. 1. Paris: The Unesco Press and la Baconnière, 1979. pp. 30-39.

Berkowitz, Gerald M. *New Broadways. Theatre Across America 1950-1980*. Totowa, New Jersey: Rowman and Littlefield, 1982.

Bhandari, Vinod, Dr. and Urmil Bhandari. "Baithaks as a Channel of Communication in Rural Area." *Journal of Family Welfare*, 19, no. 2, 1972. pp. 56-62.

Bichmann, W. "Traditional Medicine and Health Care in Africa." *Development and Cooperation*, 1984, no. 3. pp. 9-11.

Birungi, Sarah K. *A Report on AIDS Drama Competition. "The Riddle"*. 1991. Unpublished.

Bittorf, Wilhelm. "'Ngolo ist unser Gott'. Über Sexualität und AIDS in Zentralafrika." In *Der Spiegel*, no. 25, June 17th, 1991.

Björkman, Ingrid. *'Mother, Sing For Me'. People's Theatre in Kenya*. London and New Jersey: Zed Books, 1989.

Boal, Augusto. "Invisible Theatre." *Adult Education and Development*, no. 12, 1979. pp. 29-31.

Boal, Augusto. *Theater der Unterdrückten*. Frankfurt: Suhrkamp, 1989.

Boal, Augusto. *Theatre of the Oppressed*. London: Pluto Press, 1979.

Bogatyrev, Petr. *The Functions of Folk Costume in Moravian Slovakia*. The Hague, Paris: Mouton, 1971.

Breitinger, Eckhard. "Den Fortschritt inszenieren: Theaterarbeit in der Entwicklungspolitik." *Spektrum*, Universität Bayreuth, Nr. 1/90, Februar 1990. pp. 37-43.

Breitinger, Eckhard. "Popular Urban Theatre in Uganda - Between Self-Help and Self-Enrichment Strategies." *New Theatre Quarterly*, Vol. VIII, no. 31, August 1992.

Breitinger, Eckhard. "Theatre and Political Mobilisation: Case Studies from Uganda." *Matatu*, no. 11, 1994.

Brown, Winifred. *Marriage, Divorce and Inheritance. The Uganda Council of Women's Movement for Legislative Reform*. Cambridge African Monographs 10. Cambridge: African Studies Centre, 1988.

Bystrina, Ivan. *Semiotik der Kultur. Zeichen-Texte-Codes*. Tübingen: Stauffenburg Verlag, 1989.

Cabral, Amilcar. *Die Revolution der Verdammten*. Berlin: Rotbuch Verlag, 1974.

Cheney, Sheldon. *The New Movement in the Theatre*. Westport, CT: Greenwood Press, 1971.

Children and Women in Uganda. A Situation Analysis. United Nations Children's Fund. Kampala, Uganda, 1989.

Chu, Godwin C. "Group Communication and Development in Mainland China - The Functions of Social Pressure." In *Communication and Change: the Last Ten Years - and the Next*. Eds. Wilbur Schramm and Daniel Lerner. Honolulu: published for the East-West Center by the University Press of Hawaii, 1976. pp. 119-133.

Colletta, N.J. "Folk Culture and Development: Cultural Genocide or Cultural Revitalization?" *Convergence*, 10, no. 2, 1977. pp. 9-19.

Colletta, N.J. "The Use of Indigenous Culture as a Medium for Development: The Indonesian Case." *Prisma: Indonesian Journal of Social and Economic Affairs*, 1, no. 2, 1975. pp. 60-73.

Conquergood, Dwight. "Health Theatre in a Hmong Refugee Camp. Performance, Communication, and Culture." *JPR: Journal of Performance Studies*, T 119, Fall 1988. pp. 174-208.

Cook, David. "Theatre Goes to the People!" *Transition* Vol. 5, no. 25, 1966.

Cooley, Ralph E. "Codes and Contexts: An Argument For Their Description." In *Intercultural Communication Theory. Current Perspectives*. Ed. William Gudykunst. Beverly Hills, London, New Delhi: Sage Publications, 1984. pp. 241-252.

Cooper, Frederick (ed.). *Struggle for the City: Migrant Labor, Capital, and the State in Urban Africa*. Beverly Hills, London, New Delhi: Sage Publications, 1983.

Cooper, Frederick. "Who is the Populist?" *African Studies Review*, Vol. 30, no. 3, Sept. 1987.

Copeland, Roger and Marshall Cohen (eds.). *What is Dance? Readings in Theory and Criticism*. Oxford, New York, Toronto, Melbourne: Oxford University Press, 1983.

Crehan, Stewart. "Patronage, the State and Ideology in Zambian Theatre." *Journal of Southern African Studies*, Vol. 16, no. 2, June 1990. pp. 290-305.

Crow, M. and M. Etherton. "Wasan Manoma: Community Theatre in the Soba District of Kaduna State." *Savanna*, Ahmadu Bello University, Zaria, 8, 1979. pp. 6-12.

Culler, Jonathan. "Semiotics: Communication and Signification." In *Image and Code*. Ed. W. Steiner. Ann Arbor, 1981. pp. 78-84.

Cultures Vol II. Flashback. Films and History. Paris: The Unesco Press and la Baconnière, 1975.

Cultures Vol. VI. Paris: The Unesco Press and la Baconnière, 1979.

Dalfen, Charles M. "Cultural Values and Communication." In *Cultures* Vol. VI, no. 1. Paris: The Unesco Press and la Baconnière, 1979. pp. 109-114.

de Graft, J.C. "Roots in African Drama and Theatre." In *African Literature Today 8: Drama in Africa*. Ed. Eldred Durosimi Jones. London, Ibadan, Nairobi: Heinemann, 1976.

Desai, Gaurav. "Theater as Praxis: Discursive Strategies in African Popular Theater." *African Studies Review*, Vol. 33, no. 1, April 1990. pp. 65-92.

Dickson, A. "Mass Education in the Gold Coast and Togo-Land." *Mass Education Bulletin*, 1, no. 3, 1950. pp. 50-53.

Dissanayake, Wimal. "New Wine in Old Bottles; Can Folk Media Convey Modern Messages?" *Journal of Communication*, Spring 1977.

Doob, Leonard W. *Communication in Africa. A Search for Boundaries*. Westport, CT: Greenwood Press, Publishers, 1961 (reprinted 1979).

Driskell, C.B. "An Interview with Augusto Boal." *Latin American Theatre Review*, no. 8, 1975. pp. 71-78.

Dube, S.C. "Development Change and Communication in India." In *Communication and Change: The Last Ten Years - and the Next*. Eds. Wilbur Schramm and Daniel Lerner. Honolulu: published for the East-West Center by the University Press of Hawaii, 1976. pp. 98-118.

Dunlop, David Wallace. *The Economic of Uganda's Health Service System: Implications for Health and Economic Planning*. Diss. Michigan State University. Ann Arbor, Michigan: University Microfilms International, 1973.

Eco, Umberto. *Einführung in die Semiotik*. München: Wilhelm Fink Verlag, 1985.

Edwards, Nancy. "The Role of Drama in Primary Health Care." *Educational Broadcasting International*, 14, 1981, no. 2. pp. 85-89.

Egejuru, Phanuel Akubueze. *Black Writers: White Audience. A Critical Approach to African Literature*. Hicksville, New York: Exposition Press, 1988.

Ehrenhaus, Peter. "Culture and the Attribution Process: Barriers to Effective Communication." In *Intercultural Communication Theory. Current Perspectives*. Ed. William Gudykunst. Beverly Hills, London, New Delhi: Sage Publications, 1984. pp. 259-270.

Elam, Keir. *The Semiotics of Theatre and Drama*. London and New York: Methuen, 1980.

Ellingsworth, Huber W. "Adaptive Intercultural Communication." In *Intercultural Communication Theory. Current Perspectives*. Ed. William Gudykunst. Beverly Hills, London, New Delhi: Sage Publications, 1984. pp. 195-204.

Epskamp, Kees (ed.). *Education and the Development of Cultural Identity*. The Hague: CESO, 1984.

Epskamp, Kees P. *Theatre in Search of Social Change*. The Hague: CESO, 1989.

Etherton, Michael. "Trends in African Theatre." in *African Literature Today. Retrospect & Prospect*, ed. Eldred Durosimi Jones (London, Ibadan, Nairobi: Heinemann, 1979).

Etherton, Michael. *The Development of African Drama*. London, Melbourne, Sydney, Auckland, Johannesburg: Hutchinson University Library for Africa, 1982.

Eyoh, H. Ndumbe. *Hammocks To Bridges. An Experience In Theatre For Development*. Yaounde, Cameroon: BET & Co (Pub) Ltd, 1986.

Fawcett, Robin P., M.A.K. Halliday, Sydney M. Lamb, Adam Makkai (eds.). *The Semiotics of Culture and Language. Vol. 2 Language and Other Semiotic Systems of Culture*. London and Wolfeboro, N.H.: Frances Pinter (Publishers), 1984.

Fiebach, Joachim. "Offenheit und Beweglichkeit theatralischer Kommunikation in Afrika: Kulturelle Identitäten und Internationale Aspekte." In *Drama and Theatre in Africa*. Bayreuth African Studies Series 7. Ed. Eckhard Breitinger. Bayreuth: Bayreuth African Studies, 1986.

Fiebach, Joachim. *Die Toten als die Macht der Lebenden*. Wilhelmhaven: Edition Heinrichshofen, 1986.

Fischer-Lichte, Erika. "Die Zeichensprache des Theaters. Zum Problem theatralischer Bedeutungsgenerierung." In *Theaterwissenschaft heute. Eine Einführung*. Ed. Renate Möhrmann. Berlin: Dietrich Reimer Verlag, 1990. pp. 233-260.

Fischer-Lichte, Erika. "The Dramatic Dialogue - Oral or Literary Communication?" In *Semiotics of Drama and Theatre*. Ed. Aloysius van Kesteren and Herta Schmid. Amsterdam, Philadelphia: John Benjamins Publishing Company, 1984.

Fischer-Lichte, Erika. "The Theatrical Code. An Approach to the Problem." In *Multimedial Communication Vol. 2*. Ed. E. Hess-Lüttich. Tübingen: Gunter Narr Verlag, 1982.

Fischer-Lichte, Erika. "Theatre, Own and Foreign. The Intercultural Trend in Contemporary Theatre." In *The Dramatic Touch of Difference. Theatre, Own And Foreign*. Eds. E. Fischer-Lichte, Josephine Riley and Michael Gissenwehrer. Tübingen: Gunter Narr Verlag, 1990. pp. 11-22.

Fischer-Lichte, Erika. "Towards a Theory of Intercultural Performance." In *The Dramatic Touch of Difference. Theatre, Own and Foreign*. Eds. E. Fischer-Lichte, Josephine Riley and Michael Gissenwehrer. Tübingen: Gunter Narr Verlag, 1990.

Fischer-Lichte, Erika. *Semiotik des Theaters: Eine Einführung. Bd. 3. Die Aufführung als Text*. Tübingen: Gunter Narr Verlag, 1983.

Freire, Paulo. *Pedagogy of the Oppressed*. Suffolk: Penguin Books, 1972.

Fröhlich, Petra. *Das nicht-Kommerzielle amerikanische Theater*. Rheinfelden: Schäuble Verlag, 2. Auflage 1981.

Gallet, Dominique (ed.). *Dialogue pour l'identité culturelle. 1ère conférence internationale pour l'identité culturelle*. Paris: Editions Anthropos, 1982.

Gard, Robert E. and Gertrude S. Burley. *Community Theatre. Idea and Achievement*. Westport, CT: Greenwood Press, Publishers, 1975.

Gard, Robert. *Grassroots Theatre. A Search for Regional Arts in America*. Westport, CT: Greenwood Press, Publishers, 1978.

Gates, Henry Louis Jr. "The Blackness of Blackness: a Critique of the Sign and the Signifying Monkey." In *Black Literature and Literary Theory*. ed. Henry Louis Gates jr. New York and London: Methuen, 1984.

Gingyera-Pinycwa, A.G.G. *Apolo Milton Obote and His Times*. New York, London, Lagos: NOK Publishers, 1978.

Goodlad, J.R. *A Sociology of Popular Drama*. New York: Heinemann, 1971.

Gould, Julius and William L. Kolb. *A Dictionary of the Social Sciences. Compiled under the Auspices of the United Nations Educational, Scientific, and Cultural Organization*. New York: The Free Press, a Division of MacMillan publishing Co., Inc., 1988.

Grossberg, Lawrence. "Experience, Signification, and Reality: the Boundaries of Cultural Semiotics." In *Semiotica* 41-1/4 (1982), pp. 73-106.

Gudykunst, William B. Ed. *Intercultural Communication Theory. Current Perspectives*. Beverly Hills, London, New Delhi: Sage Publications, 1984.

Hagher, Iyorwuese Harry. Ed. *The Practice of Community Theatre in Nigeria*. Jos: Society of Nigerian Theatre Artists (SONTA), 1990.

Hagnell, V. "Is the Established Theatre Popular?" In *Western Popular Theatre*. Eds. David Mayer and K. Richards. London: Methuen & Co Ltd., 1977. pp. 229-238.

Halbach, Axel J. *Industriestruktur und Industrialisierungspolitik in Uganda, 1963-1972*. IFO-Institut für Wirtschaftsforschung München. Forschungsberichte der Afrikastudienstelle 50. München: Weltforum Verlag, 1974.

Hanna, Judith Lynne. *To Dance is Human. A Theory of Nonverbal Communication*. Chicago and London: The University of Chicago Press, 1987.

Hansen, Hölger Bernt and Michael Twaddle. Eds. *Changing Uganda*. London, Kampala, Athens, Nairobi: James Currey, Fountain Press, Ohio University Press, Heinemann Kenya, 1991.

Hansen, Hölger Bernt and Michael Twaddle. Eds. *Uganda Now. Between Decay & Development*. London, Athens, Nairobi: James Currey, Ohio University Press, Heinemann Kenya, 1988.

Hansen, Hölger Bernt. *Mission, Church and State in a Colonial Setting. Uganda 1890-1925*. London, Ibadan, Nairobi: Heinemann, 1984.

Hauge, Hans-Egil. *Luo Religion and Folklore*. Oslo, Bergen, Tronso: Universitetsforlaget, 1974.

Heron, George. "Uganda." In *European-Language Writing in Sub-Saharan Africa*. Ed. Albert S. Gérard. Budapest: Akdémiai Kiadó, 1986. pp. 922-948.

Hess-Lüttich, Ernest W.B. (ed.). *Multimedial Communication. Vol. 1: Semiotic Problems of its Notation*. Tübingen: Gunter Narr Verlag, 1982.

Higgs, B. "Art and National Liberation." *Young Cinema and Theatre*, 2, 1975. pp. 27-33.

Hills, Denis. *The White Pumpkin*. London: George Allen & Unwin Ltd., 1975.

Himelstein, Morgan Y. *Drama Was A Weapon. The Left-Wing Theatre in New York. 1929-1941*. Westport, CT: Greenwood Press, Publishers, 1976.

Hiß, Guido. "Zur Aufführungsanalyse". In *Theaterwissenschaft heute. Eine Einführung*. Ed. Renate Möhrmann. Berlin: Dietrich Reimer Verlag, 1990. pp. 65-80.

Hodgson, John. "Theatre in Education." *Theatre Quarterly*, Vol 1, no. 1, January-March 1971. pp. 57-60.

Hooper, Ed. *Slim*. London: The Bodley Head, 1990.

Horn, Andrew. "Individualism and Community in the Theatre of Serumaga." In *African Literature Today 12: New Writing, New Approaches*. Eds. Eldred Durosimi Jones and Eustace Palmer. London, Ibadan, Nairobi: Heinemann, 1982.

Horn, Andrew. "Uganda's Theatre - the Exiled and the Dead." In *Index on Censorship* 8 (5). London, 1979. pp. 12-15.

Horn, Andrew. "Uhuru to Amin: The Golden Decade of Theatre in Uganda." *Literary Half-Yearly*, 19, 1, 1978.

Hussein, Ibrahim. *On the Development of Theatre in East Africa*. Dissertation, Humboldt-Universität zu Berlin, Berlin, 1975.

Jakobson, Roman. *Aufsätze zur Linguistik und Poetik*. München: Nymphenburger Verlag, 1974.

Jakobson, Roman. *Semiotik: ausgewählte Texte 1919-1982*. Ed. Elmar Holenstein. Frankfurt am Main: Suhrkamp, 1988.

Janis, Irving L. "Persönlichkeitsstruktur und Beeinflußbarkeit." In *Grundfragen der Kommunikationsforschung*. Ed. Wilbur Schramm. München: Juventa Verlag, 1973. pp. 71-84.

Jefkins, Frank and Frank Ugboajah (eds.). *Communication in Industrialising Countries*. Macmillan Publishers, 1986.

Jeschke, Claudia. "Der bewegliche Blick. Aspekte der Tanzforschung." In *Theaterwissenschaft heute. Eine Einführung*. Ed. Renate Möhrmann. Berlin: Dietrich Reimer Verlag, 1990. pp. 149-164.

Jeyifo, Biodun. "The Reinvention of Theatrical Tradition: Critical Discourses on Interculturalism in the African Theatre." In *The Dramatic Touch of Difference. Theatre, Own and Foreign*. Eds. E. Fischer-Lichte, Josephine Riley and Michael Gissenwehrer. Tübingen: Gunter Narr Verlag, 1990.

Jeyifo, Biodun. *The Truthful Lie: Essays in a Sociology of African Drama*. London, Port of Spain: New Beacon Books Ltd., 1985.

Jorgensen, Jan Jelmert. *Uganda. A Modern History*. London: Croom Helm, 1981.

Jung, D. "Flowers by the Roadside...: the Relationship Between Industry and Culture in Development." *Development and Cooperation*, no. 5, 1982. pp. 23-24.

Kaahwa, Jessica. "Beyond the Pleasure Principle: The Sociological Impetus on the Theatre in Uganda: A Case Study of Country Side Youth Crude Theatre of Kibingo-Village, Bugahya Subcounty, Hoima District." Unpublished paper at the Department of Music, Dance and Drama, Makerere University, Kampala, Uganda. 1990.

Kade, Gunnar. *Die Stellung der zentralen Orte in der kulturlandschaftlichen Entwicklung Bugandas*. Frankfurt: Selbstverlag des Seminars für Wirtschaftsgeographie der Johann Wolfgang Goethe Universität Frankfurt/Main, 1969.

Kamanyi, Joanna. "A Comparative Study of Theatrical Productions in Uganda Today." Masters Thesis for Makerere University, Kampala/Uganda, 1978.

Karugire, S.R. *A Political History of Uganda*. Nairobi, London: Heinemann Educational Books, 1980.

Karugire, S.R. *The Roots of Instability in Uganda* (Kampala: The New Vision Printing and Publishing Co-operation, 1988).

Kasfir, Nelson. *The Shrinking Political Arena. Participation and Ethnicity in African Politics, with a Case Study of Uganda*. Berkeley, Los Angeles, London: University of California Press, 1976.

Katz, Elihu. "Can Authentic Cultures Survive New Media?" *Journal of Communication*, Spring 1977.

Katz, Elihu. "Die Verbreitung neuer Ideen und Praktiken." In *Grundfragen der Kommunikationsforschung*. Ed. Wilbur Schramm. München: Juventa Verlag, 1973. pp. 99-116.

Kazacoff, George. *Dangerous Theatre*. New York, Bern, Frankfurt am Main, Paris: Peter Lang, 1989.

Kennedy, Scott. *In Search of African Theatre*. New York: Charles Scribner's Sons, 1973.

Kerr, David. "Didactic Theatre in Africa." *Harvard Educational Review 51*, no. 1, 1981. pp. 145-155.

Khan, Akhter Hamee. "The Comilla Experience in Bangladesh - My Lessons in Communication." In *Communication and Change: The Last Ten Years - and the Next*. Eds. Wilbur Schramm and Daniel Lerner. Honolulu: published for the East-West Center by the University Press of Hawaii, 1976. pp. 67-82.

Kidd, R. "From Outside In to Inside Out; The Benue Workshop on Theatre for Development." *Media in Development*, March 1983.

Kidd, R. "Liberation or Domestication: Popular Theatre and Non-Formal Education in Africa." *Young Cinema and Theatre*, no. 4, 1982. pp. 8-17.

Kidd, R. "Popular Theatre and Popular Struggle in Kenya: the Story of Kamiriithu." *Race and Class*, Vol. XXIV, 3, 1983.

Kidd, R. and M. Byram. "Demystifying Pseudo-Freirian Development. The Case of Laedza Batanani." *Community Development Journal*, 1712, 1982. pp. 91-105.

Kidd, R. and M. Byram. "Popular Theatre and Development: a Botswana Case Study." *Convergence*, 10, no. 2, 1977. pp. 20-30.

Kidd, R. and M. Byram. "Popular Theatre as a Tool for Community Education in Botswana." *Assignment Children: a Journal Concerned with Children, Women and Youth in Development* (Unicef), no. 44, 1978. pp. 35-65.

Kidd, Ross. "Plays for Farmers: Popular Drama Workshops in Northern Nigeria. Stage Two: from Outside-In to Inside-Out." *Théâtre International*, no. 6, 2, 1982. pp. 25-44.

Kincaid, D. Lawrence and June Ock Yum. "The Needle and the Ax - Communication and Development in a Korean Village." In *Communication and Change: The Last Ten Years - and the Next*. Eds. Wilbur Schramm and Daniel Lerner. Honolulu: published for the East-West Center by the University Press of Hawaii, 1976. pp. 83-97.

Kisense, Daniel Isiko. "Theatre and Drama in Uganda. Drama Groups and their Activities." Unpublished paper, Department of Music, Dance and Drama, Makerere University, Kampala, Uganda, 1991.

Kiwanuka, Semakula. *Amin and the Tragedy of Uganda*. München and London: Weltforum Verlag, 1979.

Klein, Eberhard C. *Sozialer Wandel in Kiteezi/Buganda*. München: Weltforum Verlag, 1969.

Knappert, Jan. *Bantu Myths and Other Tales*. Leiden: E.J. Brill, 1977.

Kranich. Uganda Nachrichten. no. 7, May 1992.

Kranich. Uganda Nachrichten. no. 1, no year.

Kristeva, Julia. *Die Revolution der poetischen Sprache*. Frankfurt: Suhrkamp, 1978.

Kruse, W. "The Barefoot Doctor: a Solution to Health Needs?" *Development and Cooperation*, 1978, no. 3. pp. 13-15.

Lange, Roderyk. *The Nature of Dance. An Anthropological Perspective*. London: MacDonald & Evans Ltd., 1975.

Larlham, Peter. *Black Theater, Dance and Ritual in South Africa*. Ann Arbor, Michigan: Umi Research Press, 1985.

Lent, J.A. "Grassroots Rennaissance: the Increasing Importance of Folk Media in Third World Nations." *Asian Folklore Studies 39*, no. 2, 1980, pp. 145-162.

Leshoai, B. "Tanzania: Socialist Theatre." *New Theatre Magazine*, 12, no. 2, 1972. pp. 22-23.

Leysen, Luc. "Die Kinder der Seuche. AIDS-Waisen in Afrika." Report shown in ARD, 4.2.91. (script by WDR).

Lihamba, Amandina. "Health and The African Theatre." *Review of African Political Economy*, 36, 1986. pp. 35-40.

Lotman, Ju. M. *Die Struktur literarischer Texte*. München: Wilhelm Fink Verlag, 1986.

Low, D.A. *The Mind of Buganda. Documents of the Modern History of an African Kingdom*. London, Ibadan, Nairobi: Heinemann, 1971.

Low, Donald A. *Buganda in Modern History*. Berkeley and Los Angeles: University of California Press, 1971.

Mac Cannel, Dean. "Ethnosemiotics." In *Semiotics of Culture*. Eds. Irene Portis Winner and Jean Umiker Sebeok. The Hague, Paris, New York: Mouton Publishers, 1979. pp. 149-171.

Mair, Lucy, P. Mair. *Magie im schwarzen Erdteil*. München: Kindlers Universitätsbibliothek, 1969.

Makagiansar, Makaminian. Reading the Report of the Director General of Unesco. *Cultures*, Vol. VI (Paris: the Unesco Press and la Baconnière, 1979).

Mamdani, Mahmood. *Politics and Class Formation in Uganda*. New York and London: Monthly Review Press, 1976.

Martin, David. *General Amin*. London: Faber & Faber, 1974.

Martin, William. "Theatre as Social Education." *Theatre Quarterly*, Vol. II, no. 8, Oct.-Dec. 1972. pp. 18-26.

Marvin, Richard. *Land or Wages. The Evaluation of Occupational and Residential Alternatives by the Rural Basoga*. IFO-Institut für Wirtschaftsforschung München. Afrika-Studien 101. München, London: Weltforum Verlag, 1978.

Mbiti, John. *African Religions and Philosophy*. London: Heinemann, 1982.

Mbogo, Emmanuel. *Pre-Capitalist - Pre-Colonial Theater in East Africa: Kenya, Uganda and Tanzania*. Dissertation, Humboldt-Universität zu Berlin, Berlin, 1985.

Mbowa, Rose. "Ugandan Literature," Ringvorlesung, Bayreuth University, July 11th 1991.

Mbughuni, L.A. "Old And New Drama From East Africa. A Review of the Works of Four Contemporary Dramatists: Rebecca Njau, Ebrahim Hussein, Peninah Muhando and Ngugi." In *African Literature Today 8*. London, Ibadan, Nairobi, Lusaka: Heinemann, 1976.

Mbughuni, L.A. "The Development of English Drama in East Africa. A Study of the Emergence of New Trends of Modern Theatre and Drama." In *The Writing of East and Central Africa*. Ed. G.D. Killam. London, Ibadan, Nairobi: Heinemann, 1984.

McGrath, John. *A Good Night Out*. London: Methuen, 1981.

McPherson, Margaret. "Plays and People: An Examination of Three Ugandan Dramatists: Byron Kawadwa, John Ruganda and Robert Serumaga." Paper presented to the Makerere Golden Jubilee Writers' Workshop, University of Nairobi, December 18th-23rd, 1972, p. 4.

Meggle, Georg. *Grundbegriffe der Kommunikation*. Berlin, New York: Walter de Gruyter, 1981.

Melady, Thomas and Margaret. *Idi Amin Dada: Hitler in Africa*. Kansas City: Sheed Andrews and McMeel, 1977.

Mellgren, T. "Augusto Boal's Theatre of the Oppressed." *Canadian Theatre Review*, 19, 1978. pp. 108-114.

Mensah, Augustine K. *Autoritätskonzept und Autoritätswandel in Ghana, Nigeria und Uganda*. Dissertation, München, 1970.

Michalsky, Y. "The 'Active Spectator' Takes the Floor: An Interview with Augusto Boal." *Yale Theatre*, vol. 12, no. 1, 1980. pp. 14-18.

Michaud, Guy (ed.). *Identités collectives et relations inter-culturelles*. Bruxelles: Editions Complexe, 1978.

Mirembe, Mercy. "The Influence of Ugandan Folklore on Ugandan Theatre." MA-thesis, Makerere University, Kampala/Uganda, 1990, unpublished.

Mkanju. "Dramatising the pain of AIDS." *The Sunday Nation* (Kenya), August 25, 1991.

Mlama, Penina Muhando. *Culture and Development. The Popular Theatre Approach in Africa*. Uppsala: The Scandinavian Institute of African Studies, 1991.

Möhrmann, Renate Ed. *Theaterwissenschaft heute. Eine Einführung*. Berlin: Dietrich Reimer Verlag, 1990.

Mowlana, Hamid. "Mass Media and Culture: Toward an Integrated Theory." In *Intercultural Communication Theory. Current Perspectives*. Ed. William Gudykunst. Beverly Hills, London, New Delhi: Sage Publications, 1984. pp. 149-170.

Muganga, Jonathan. "Theatre for Development in Uganda. The Nattyole Experience." (Ministry of Health (Uganda) Health Education Division) 1990, unpublished research report.

Mugizi, Patrick. "Nakivubo cries, laughs, and mocks Lutaaya." *Weekly Topic* (Uganda), November 8, 1989.

Mukarovsky, Jan. *Kapitel aus der Ästhetik*. Frankfurt: Suhrkamp Verlag, 1982.

Müller, Klaus E. *Das magische Universum der Identität*. Frankfurt, New York: Campus Verlag, 1987.

Müller-Doohm, Stefan and Klaus Neumann (eds.). *Medienforschung und Kulturanalyse. Ein Werkstattbericht*. Oldenburg: Bibliotheks- und Informationssystem der Universität Oldenburg, 1989.

Multimedial Communication. Vol. II: Theatre Semiotics. Tübingen: Gunter Narr Verlag.

Mwaniki, H.S.K. *Categories and Substance of Embu Traditional Songs and Dances*. Nairobi: Kenya Literature Bureau, 1986.

Mwansa, Dickson M. "Theatre as a Tool for Communication." *Ifda dossier*, no. 42, 1984. pp. 23-32.

Ngugi wa Mirii. "Literacy for and by the People: Kenya's Kamiriithu Project." *Convergence*, 8, no. 4, 1980. pp. 55-61.

Ngugi, wa Thiong'o. "Women in Cultural Work: the Fate of Kamiriithu People's Theatre Kenya." *Development Dialogue*, Vol. 1-2. The Dag Hammars-Kjöld Foundation, Uppsala, 1983.

Obudho, R.A. and Salah El-Shaks. *Development of Urban Systems in Africa*. New York: Praeger, 1979.

Omana-Otunnu, Amii. *Politics and the Military in Uganda, 1890-1985*. Oxford: Macmillan Press/St. Antony's College, 1987.

P'Chong, Cliff Lubwa. "Where From, and Where To Now?" Masters Thesis in Education of the University of Durham, 1987; unpublished.

Pasquali, Antonio. "Understanding Communication or the Media?" In *Cultures* Vol. VI, no. 3. Paris: the Unesco Press and la Baconnière, 1979, pp. 11-28.

Pickering, A.K. "Village Drama in Ghana." *Fundamental and Adult Education*, no. 4, 1957. pp. 178-183.

Pörtner, Paul. *Spontanes Theater. Erfahrungen Konzepte*. Köln: Kiepenheuer & Witsch, 1972.

Poyatos, Fernando. *New Perspectives in Nonverbal Communication. Studies in Cultural Anthropology, Social Psychology, Linguistics, Literature, and Semiotics*. Oxford, New York, Toronto, Sydney, Paris, Frankfurt: Pergamon Press, 1983.

Quilligan, Maureen. *The Language of Allegory. Defining the Genre*. Ithaca and London: Cornell University Press, 1979.

Rewar, Walter. "Notes for a Typology of Culture." In *Semiotica* 18, 4. The Hague, Paris: Mouton Publishers, 1976. pp. 361-378.

Richards, Sandra. "Toward a Populist Nigerian Theatre: The Plays of Femi Osofisan." *New Theatre Quarterly* 3, 11, 1987.

Roberg, Dietmar. *Theater muß wie Fußball sein*. Berlin: Rotbuchverlag, 1981.

Rokeach, Milton. *The Nature of Human Values*. New York: Free Press, 1973.

Royce, Anya Peterson. *The Anthropology of Dance*. Bloomington and London: Indiana University Press, 1977.

Rusch, Walter. *Klassen und Staat in Buganda vor der Kolonialzeit*. Veröffentlichungen des Museums für Völkerkunde zu Leipzig. Heft 25. Berlin: Akademie Verlag, 1975.

Rwagacuzi, Faustin. *A History of Ugandan Disunity with Special Attention to Buganda from the Middle of the Nineteenth Century to the First Years of Independence in 1962*. Dissertation, Claremont Graduate School. Ann Arbor, Michigan: University Microfilms International, 1981.

Ryle, John. "A Dance of Death." *TLS*, April 27-May 3, 1990.

Sarbaugh, L.E. and Nobleza Asuncion-Lande. "Theory Building in Intercultural Communication: Synthesizing the Action Caucus." In *Intercultural Communication Theory. Current Perspectives*. Ed. William Gudykunst. Beverly Hills, London, New Delhi: Sage Publications, 1984. pp. 45-62.

Satyamurthy, T.V. *The Political Development of Uganda: 1900-1986*. Hants/England a. Brookfield, Vermont/U.S.A.: Gower, 1986.

Sawant, G.K. "Shadow Play: a Tool for the Dissemination of Ideas." *Adult Education and Development*, no. 23, 1984. pp. 109-112.

Schechner, Richard and Willa Appel (eds.). *By Means of Performance. Intercultural Studies of Theatre and Ritual*. Cambridge, New York, Port Chester, Melbourne, Sydney: Cambridge University Press, 1990.

Schechner, Richard. *Between Theater and Anthropology*. Philadelphia: University of Pennsylvania Press, 1985.

Schmid, Josef. *Der Kulturbegriff als analytisches und ideologiekritisches Instrument der Soziologie*. Dissertation, Ludwig-Maximilians-Universität zu München, München, 1974.

Schramm, Wilbur (ed.). *Grundfragen der Kommunikationsforschung*. München: Juventa Verlag, 1973.

Schramm, Wilbur and Daniel Lerner (eds.). *Communication and Change. The Last Ten Years - and the Next*. Honolulu: published for the East-West Center by the University Press of Hawaii, 1976.

Schramm, Wilbur. "An Overview of the Past Decade." In *Communication and Change. The Last Ten Years - and the Next*. Eds. Wilbur Schramm and Daniel Lerner. Honolulu: published for the East-West Center by the University Press of Hawaii, 1976. pp. 1-6.

Sempebwa, Joshua W. *African Traditional Moral Norms and Their Implication for Christianity. A Case Study of Ganda Ethics*. St. Augustin: Steyler Verlag, 1983.

Sempebwa, Joshua W. *The Ontological and Normative Structure in the Social Reality of a Bantu Society. A Systematic Study of Ganda Ontology and Ethics*. Dissertation, Ruprecht-Karl-Universität Heidelberg, Heidelberg, 1978.

Senasi, Benjamin. "Ugandans Not Scared by AIDS." *Weekly Topic* (Uganda), March 7, 1982.

Shack, William A. and Elliott P. Skinner (eds.). *Strangers in African Societies*. Berkeley, Los Angeles, London: University of California Press, 1979.

Shank, T. "The Theatre and Social Change: Principles and Techniques." *Young Cinema and Theatre*, 1, 1977. pp. 3-12.

Siné, Babacar. "Cultural Dynamics and New Communication Techniques in Black Africa." In *Cultures* Vol. VI, no. 3. Paris: The Unesco Press and la Baconnière, 1979, pp. 74-88.

Smith, George Ivan. *Ghosts of Kampala*. London: Weidenfeld and Nicolson, 1980.

Spruck, Stefan. "Das Land der leeren Dörfer. Aidstod in Uganda." In *Weltjournal* Nr. 22 - 4.12.91. Report shown in NDR.

Szanto, George H. *Theater and Propaganda*. Austin: University of Texas Press, 1978.

Tafoya, Dennis W. "The Roots of Conflict: A Theory and Typology." In *Intercultural Communication Theory. Current Perspectives*. Ed. William Gudykunst. Beverly Hills, London, New Delhi: Sage Publications, 1984. pp. 205-240.

Tandon, R. "The Interlinkages between Primary Health Care and Adult Education." *Convergence*, 15, 1982, no. 2. pp. 3-13.

Taylor, D. "Living Images: the Politics of Culture." *New Internationalist*, no. 98, 1981. pp. 7-9.

Tehranian, Majid. "Communication and International Development: Some Theoretical Considerations." In *Cultures* Vol. VI, no. 3. Paris: The Unesco Press and la Baconnière, 1979, pp. 29-37.

Turner, Victor. "Forms of Symbolic Action: Introduction. In *"Forms of Symbolic Action." Proceedings of the 1969 Annual Spring Meeting of the American Ethnological Society*, Ed. R.F. Spencer. Seattle, London, 1969.

Turner, Victor. *Vom Ritual zum Theater. Der Ernst des menschlichen Spiels*. Frankfurt, New York: Edition Qumran im Campus Verlag, 1989.

Tzeng, Oliver C.S., C.J. Duvall, Roger Ware, Robert Neel and Robert Fortier. "Subjective Intergroup Distances of Blacks and Whites." In *Interethnic Communication. Current Research*. Ed. Young Yun KIM. Newbury Park, Beverly Hills, London, New Delhi: SAGE Publications, 1986.

Uspensky et. al. "Theses on the Semiotic Study of Culture (As Applied to Slavic Texts)." In *Structure of Texts and Semiotics of Culture*. Eds. Jan van der Eng and Mojmir Grygor. The Hague, Paris: Mouton, 1973. pp. 1-28.

Wadulo, Geoffrey. "'Theatre for Development' in Uganda." 1990, unpublished research report.

Waldmann, Günter. *Kommunikationsästhetik 1. Die Ideologie der Erzählform*. München: Wilhelm Fink Verlag, 1976.

Weidig, Jutta. *Tanz-Ethnologie. Einführung in die völkerkundliche Sicht des Tanzes*. Ahrensburg bei Hamburg: Verlag Ingrid Czwalina, 1984.

Werner, Alice. *Myths and Legends of the Bantu*. London: Frank Cass & Co. Ltd., 1968.

Werner, D. and B. Bower. "Village Theatre: the Importance of Breast-Feeding." *Adult Education and Development*, 1983, no. 20. pp. 71-79.

Whitman, Jon. *Allegory. The Dynamics of An Ancient and Medieval Technique*. Oxford: Clarendon Press, 1987.

Winner, Irene Portis and Jean Umiker Sebeok (eds.). *Semiotics of Culture*. The Hague, Paris, New York: Mouton Publishers, 1979.

Winner, Irene Portis and Thomas G. Winner. "The Semiotics of Cultural Texts." In *Semiotica* 18, 2, The Hague, Paris: Mouton Publishers, 1976. pp. 101-156.

Winner, Irene Portis. "Ethnicity, Modernity, and Theory of Culture Texts." In *Semiotics of Culture*. Eds. Irene Portis Winner and Jean Umiker Sebeok. The Hague, Paris, New York: Mouton Publishers, 1979. pp.103-147.

Winner, Thomas G. "Some Fundamental Concepts Leading to a Semiotics of Culture: A Historical Overview." In *Semiotics of Culture*. Eds. Irene Portis Winner and Jean Umiker Sebeok. The Hague, Paris, New York: Mouton Publishers, 1979. pp. 75-83.

Wooding, Dan and Ray Barnett. *Uganda Holocaust*. Grand Rapids, Michigan: Zondervan Publishing House, 1980.

Wright, A.C.A. "Some Notes on Acoli Religious Ceremonies," *Uganda Journal*, III, 3, January, 1936.

Zima, Peter V. *Textsoziologie. Eine kritische Einführung*. Stuttgart: J.B. Metzlersche Verlagsbuchhandlung, 1980.

Ziolkowski, Janusz. "Cultural Dimension of Development." In *Cultures* Vol. VI, no. 1. Paris: The Unesco Press and la Baconnière, 1979, pp. 17-29.

Bayreuth African Studies Series
Available Titles:

1 The Sudan: Ethnicity and National Cohesion
- Ethnicity, Regionalism and National Cohesion in the Sudan
- National Versus Regional: Methodological Problems in the Study of Nationalism and Nation Building in the Sudan
- The Dynamics of Ethnic Identification in Northern Dafur, Sudan

Price per title: DM 12,-

2 Towards African Authenticity
- The First African Novels in French: A Problem of Authenticity
- The Question of Ethnic Traditions Within a National Literature: The Example of Nigeria
- Early 20th Century Swahili Prose Narrative Structure and Some Aspects of Swahili Ethnicity
- The Development of Sierra Leone Krio

Price per title: DM 12,-

3 Littératures Africaines francophones
- Oralité, écriture et le problème de l'identité culturelle en Afrique
- Le concept de littérature nationale
- Au coeur de la littérature negro-africaine d'écriture française:

Price per title: DM 12,-

4 Approaches to African Identity
- Identity and the Political Economy of Islamic Conversion in Africa
- Difficultés de la notion d'universalité latérale
- Identity - Some Encouragements from a Psychological Perspective
- Identität in Gesetzgebung und Rechtsprechung in Afrika
- Identity and Socio-Economic Change in Nigeria - An Overview

Price per title: DM 12,- (out of print)

5 Language and Education in Africa
- Al-Hajj Sa'ad Umar Touré and Islamic Education Reform in Mali
- Conflicting Interests which Influence Hausa Women
- Sciences, techniques et cultures africaines
- English in Tanzanian Education
- Multilingualism and Language Policy in Sierra Leone

Price per title: DM 12,- (out of print)

6 Literature and African Identity
- Xenophobia and Class Consciousness in Recent Africa
- Literature and African Identity: The Example of Ayi Kwei Armah
- Is There a Nigerian Literature ?
- Le thème de l'identité culturelle dans le roman africain francophone

Price per title: DM 12,-

7 Drama and Theatre in Africa
- Offenheit und Beweglichkeit theatralischer Kommunikation in Afrika: Kulturelle Identitäten und internationale Aspekte
- Les origines d'un théâtre national africain: Le cas nigerian
- Radical Conservatism in Yoruba Popular Plays

Price per title: DM 12,-

8 Interviews avec des écrivains africains francophones

Interviews avec
- René Philombe
- Dono Ly Sangaré
- Amadou Koné
- Bernard Zadi Zaourou
- Jean Marie Adiaffi

Price per title: DM 12,-

9 Perspectives on African Music
- Afrikanische Musik, Ideologischer Kolonialismus und Identitätskrise der Zöglingsgeneration 1945-1970
- Musical Traditions, Islam and Cultural Identity in the Sudan
- Ebenezer Calender - An Appraisal
- Transcription and Translation of Calender's Repertoire List
- The Language and Content of Nigerian Popular Music
- Jambo Records and the Promotion of Popular Music in East Africa.

Price per title: DM 18,50

10 Douala 1893 - La Revolte des esclaves mercenaires

by **Adjai Paulin Oloukpona-Yinnon**

Price per title: DM 12,-

11 African and Western Legal Systems in Contact
- The Machinery of Justice in Nigeria
- The Impact of English Law Concepts on the Administration of Islamic Law in Nigeria
- The Changing Role of the Extended Family

Price per title: DM 12,-

12 Three Yoruba Artists
- Twins Seven-Seven
- Ademola Onibonokuta
- Muraina Oyelami

Price per title: DM 12,- (out of print)

13 Patterns of Language Knowledge and Language Use in Ngamiland in Botswana

by **Rainer Vossen**

Price per title: DM 12,-

14 KULANKULA - Interviews with Writers from Malawi and Lesotho
- Aubrey Kalitera
- Ken Lipenga
- Anthony Nazombe
- Njabulo S. Ndebele
- David Rubadiri

Price per title: DM 12,-

15 English in East and Central Africa I
- English in East Africa: Theoretical, methodological and practical issues
- Attitudes towards English among Kenyan students
- 'Non-Problematic Zambianisms' and their implications for the teaching of English in Zambia
- Second-language varieties across the Indian Ocean

Price per title: DM 12,-

16 Essays on Music in Africa 2
- Jùjú, Fújì and the Intercultural Aspects of Modern Yoruba Popular Music
- Concepts of Neo-African Music as Manifested in the Yoruba Folk Opera
- My Approach to Neo-African Music Theatre
- Intercultural Expressions in Neo-African Art Music

Price per title: DM 29,- (out of print)

17 New Religious Movements and Society in Nigeria
- The Quest for Identity in African New Religious Movements
- New Religious Movements and the Nigerian Social Order
- Spiritual Church Participation as a Survival Strategy
- Nationalistic Motifs in a Nigerian New Religious Movement

Price per title: DM 12,-

18 Linguistics in the Service of Africa
Edited by **Josef Schmied**
- Linguistics in the service of Africa: a retrospective view
- Researching into second language use and usage: with special reference to SeTswana in Ngamiland, Botswana
- Lexical problems of English in Africa
- Research into English and African languages in Nigeria
- A Corpus of East African English: prospects and problems
- English and African languages: excerpts from a discussion

Price per title: DM 12,-

19/20 Littérature et Politique en Afrique noire
by **Koffi Anyinefa**
Price per title: DM 39,-

21/22 Yoruba Drumming. The Dundun Tradition
by **Akin Euba**
Price per title: DM 59,-

23 Le Champs littéraire togolais
Edité par **János Riesz** et **Alain Ricard**
- Le champ littéraire togolais
- Génération Eyadema. Littérature populaire et littérature d'élite
- Firminger, Nachtigal, Zöller: trois témoins de la naissance du Togo (1884). A la recherche des premiers documents écrits de l'histoire togolais
- Sources allemandes sur l'histoire du Togo - 1884-1914
- Dietrich Westermann: pionnier de la recerche sur la culture ewe
- Entre littérature et propagande: les "Belles Lettres" coloniales allemandes sur le Togo
- Quand la littérature enjambe la frontière: "Amour de Féticheuse (au Dahomey et) au Togo" de Félix Couchoro
- Des écrivains et des langues: les Ewe qui écrivent
- La presse togolaise avant l'indépendance
- Le Togo diglossique? Proposition pour l'analyse d'une conscience linguistique au Sud du Togo
- Le palimpseste de l'écriture ouest-africaine francophone
- Agbebada meets Mister Tameklor. Un sujet, deux pièces de théâtre, trois générations: changement et continuité dans la société ewe
- La poésie togolaise en langue française. Réflexions sur l'"Anthologie de la poésie togolaise"

Price per title: DM 29,-

24 English in East and Central Africa 2
edited by **Josef Schmied**
- Deviation and language awareness in Kenyan popular literature
- Richer or rotten? A study of borrowing from English to Dholuo
- Establishing educational bilingual programmes in Tanzania: an alternative option
- Comprehension and sentence complexity in Tanzanian classrooms
- Assessing second language learner proficiency in Zambia
- Some grammatical sign-posts in Cameroon Standard English
- The role of English in education in Southern Africa

Price per title: DM 15,-

25 Akin Euba - An Introduction to the Life and Music of a Nigerian Composer
by **Joshua Uzoigwe**
Price per title: DM 19,80

26 Gros-Plan sur les femmes en Afrique / Afrikanische Frauen im Blick / Focus on Women in Africa
edited by **Gudrun Ludwar-Ene** and **Mechthild Reh**
- "Homme Nénuphar" - Discours amoureux et discours identitaire dans le poème "Latérite" de Véronique Tadjo
- *Kwantacce*, the 'Sleeping Pregnancy', a Hausa Concept
- The Social Relationships of Female and Male Migrants in Calabar, Nigeria: Rural Versus Urban Connections
- Industrieunternehmerinnen - Modell für einen Weg aus der ökonomischen Marginalisierung nigerianischer Frauen?
- Zur Problematik der Grundschulbildung für Mädchen in den ländlichen Regionen Nordkameruns
- Les activités des enfants dans les ménages abidjanais: A propos de la fonction socialisante du travail
- Macht und Religiöse Vielfalt im Norden Ugandas
- Protection of Widows and Administration of Customary Estates in Zambian Courts

Price per title: DM 29,-

27 Survey of Zimbabwean Writers. Educational and Literary Careers
by **Flora Veit-Wild**
Price per title: DM 29,-

28 Konflikte im kolonialen Alltag
by **Norbert Aas** and **Harald Sippel**
Price per title: DM 14,80

29 Intercultural Music I
edited by **Cynthia Tse Kimberlin** and **Akin Euba**
Price per title: about DM 39,-

30 Anglophone Cameroon Writing
edited by **Nalova Lyonga**, **Bole Butake** and **Eckhard Breitinger**
Price per title: DM 29,-

31 Theatre and Performance in Africa: Intercultural Perspectives
edited by **Eckhard Breitinger**
- Theatre for Development or Live and Let Live
- Designing a Multi-Ethnic Theatrical Idiom: Rose Mbowa´s *Mother Uganda and Her Children*
- Identity and Social Contexts of Cultural Transfer in Black Drama
- Patterns of Communication: Wole Soyinka´s *Death and the King´s Horseman...*
- Masquerade Elements on the Stage Today
- Perspectives in Popular Theatre: Orality as a Definition of New Realities
- The Dramatist at Work: My Theatre Work is Aimed at the Urbano-Politico-Bureaucratic Elite in Cameroon
- Another Theatre of the Absurd
- Theatre at Nigerian Universities
- Artists Under Siege: Theatre and the Dictatorial Regimes in Uganda
- "... satirizing those aspects of our life we don´t approve of" - A View of the "Dark Comedies" from the Townships
- Junction Avenue Theatre Company´s *Tooth and Nail*. The State of ´Interregnum´ and New Theatre Forms in South Africa
- Song, Story and Nation: Women as Singers and Actresses in Zimbabwe
- The Quest for a New Literary Idiom in Nigeria´s TV-Plays
- Children´s Theatre in Cameroon: Some Experiences

Price per title: DM 39,-

32 The Novels of Nuruddin Farah
by **Derek Wright**
Price per title: DM 29,- (US $21.50, £ 11.95)
cloth: DM 44,90 (US $ 34.50, £ 19.90)

33 Échanges Franco-Allemands sur l´Afrique
edited by **János Riesz & Hélène d´Almeida-Topor**
Price per title: DM 39,- (£ 16.95, US $ 27.95)
- La diffusion du pain en Afrique noire
- Is there "Land Shortage" in the Usambara Mountains / Tanzania?
- Santé et colinisation: épidémiologie et démographie en AEF et au Cameroun

- Contribution à l´étude des clivages sociaux dans le royaume de Jaara (Mali, Mauritanie) du XVIe siècle
- Le statut très particulier des "bâtards" de Rehoboth en Afrique Allemande du Sud-Ouest, ou la peur du métissage
- Ville en Afrique ou ville d´Afrique? Quelques remarques sur le fait urbain dans le "pool" congolais précolonial
- Micro-projets et associations de solidarité internationale: conditions de réussite et facteurs de blocage
- Position de recherche - Entre le champ, la cuisine et le marché. Enquête sur la gestion paysanne des vivres en Afrique occidentale
- Creolization and Pidginization as Categories odf Cultural Differentiation in Freetown
- De la littérature orale dans les revues coloniales: l´exemple de *Notes Africaines*
- Une méthode d´approche du marché de l´automobile en Côte d´Ivoire de 1945 à 1980
- L´Afrique dans les relations frano-allemandes entre les deux guerres: du contexte historique aux textes littéraires
- Islamic Learning and "Western Education" in Nigeria: Concepts, Institutions, and Conflicts
- L´étrange messe du père Kamara
- Jean-Paul Sartre, Simone de Beauvoir et l´Afrique
- Champ littéraire hétérogène: quelques observations sur la littérature congolaise à partir de l´oeuvre de Sony Labou Tansi et du roman latino-américain dit du "boom"
- Les enfants de Saanɛ et de Kontoron: à propos des chasseurs du Manden

34 **Contemporary Relativism with Special Reference to Culture and Africa**
by **Ernest Beyaraza**
Price per title: DM 39,- (£ 16.95, US $ 27.95)

35 **Aids-Education through Theatre. Case Studies from Uganda**
by **Marion Frank**
Price per title: DM 39,- (£ 16.95, US $ 27.95)

36 **Theatre for Development - Le théâtre au service du développement**
Bilingual edition. In cooperation with GtZ.
(with 20 full colour photographs)
edited by **Eckhard Breitinger**
Price per title: DM 24,80 (£ 9.99, US $ 17.90)
- Theatre for Development: A Strategy for Communication and Conscientisation
- Popularising Projects and Programms
- The Groups and their Plays

37 **Author, Publisher and Gikuyu Nationalist: The Life and Writings of Gakaara wa Wanjau**
In cooperation with IFRA, Nairobi
by **Cristiana Pugliese**
Price per title: DM 39,- (£ 16.95, US $ 27.95)

38 **Sénégal-Forum: Histoire et Littérature**
edited by **Papa Samba Diop**
Price per title: DM 39,- (£ 16.95, US $ 27.95)
- De l´oralité à l´écriture: transcription et création
- La quête de l´ancêtre historique: le paradigme de Sunjata dans les traditions orales du Sahel (XIIe-XIXe siècles)
- Les genres narratifs et les phénomènes intertextuels dans l´espace soudanais
- Solidarité familiale et réussite individuelle dans la société sénégalaise
- *L´Aventure ambiguë*: la folie ou le refus de l´ambiguïté
- De l´épopée au mythe: le *Chaka* de Senghor
- Effets de réel, effets étranges. Une écriture de la diversité dans *Signare Anna* de Tita Mandeleau
- La filiation mythique et historique entre ly royauté du Tekruur et celle de Wolof
- Le Jihaad omarien dans le royaume de Segu (1859-1861)
- Interdisciplinary Approaches to the pre-16th century History of Casamance and Northern Guiné-Bissau
- Lamine Senghor (1889-1927), précurseur de la prose nationaliste négro-africaine
- Traduire le *way*. Le chant selon Senghor
- "Le dernier voyage du Négrier Sirius": le roman dans le roman *Le Docker Noir* (1956) d´Ousmane Sembène
- Essai de typologie des chants soninke: contexte de production et approche thématique
- Le Sénégal dans les encyclopédies allemandes
- Entretien avec Khadi Fall
- Entretien avec Yunus Jeng
- Deux figures héroïques de l´aire mande: le *ceddo* et le *nana*
- Acculturation coloniale et pédagogie interculturelle: l´oeuvre de Georges Hardy

39 **Uganda: The Literary Landscape**
edited by **Rose Mbowa & Eckhard Breitinger**
Price per title: DM 39,- (£ 16.95, US $ 27.95)
(forthcoming)

Prices do not include postage.
ALSO AVAILABLE:

Transition and Continuity of Identity in East Africa and Beyond - In Memoriam David Miller.
Edited by **Elisabeth Linnebuhr** (517 pp., illustrations), DM 59,-

Subsistence Cultivation, Market Production and Agricultural Development in Ruvuma Region, Southern Tanzania.
by Doris Schmied (208 pp.), DM 29,-

Frankophones Theater im Senegal. Seine Herausbildung und Entwicklung von den Anfängen bis zur Gegenwart.
by **Günter Bielemeier** (331 pp.), DM 39,-

The Sociolinguistic Impact of Kiswahili on Ethnic Community Languages in Tanzania: A Case Study of Ekinata.
by **Rugatiri D. K. Mekacha** (260 pp.), DM 29,-

Aspects of Interphonology: The Study of Kenyan Learners of Swahili.
by **Paul Muthoka Musau** (236 pp.), DM 29,-

Erbrecht an Grund und Boden in Benin.
by **Ahonagnon Noel Gbaguidi** (243 pp.), DM 29,-

Ntoota Kimbuzi. Koongo - Zayidi - Ngola.
by **Miabeto Ladi** (55 pp.), DM 10,-

Arbeit und Beruf bei Handwerkern der Bakiga in Uganda.
by **Georg Eduard Heidenreich** (237 pp.), DM 39,-

Orders for all titles to:
Eckhard Breitinger, University of Bayreuth, D-95440 Bayreuth, Germany
Tel. (0)921 - 55-3571; Fax: (0)921 - 55-3627; E-mail: Eckhard.Breitinger@uni-bayreuth.de